WITHOUT
CHILD

*A Compassionate
Look
at Infertility*

Martha Stout

Harold Shaw Publishers
Wheaton, Illinois

for Kathleen Murphy Jones

ISBN 0-87788-910-4

Library of Congress Cataloging-in-Publication Data

Stout, Martha G.
    Without child : a compassionate look at infertility / Martha Stout.
        p. cm.
        ISBN 0-87788-910-4
        1. Infertility, Female—Psychological aspects. 2. Miscarriage—Psychological aspects. 3. Adoption—Psychological aspects. 4. Christian life—1960- I. Title.
        RG201.S76 1990
        618.1'78'0019—dc20   89-29867
                                                            CIP

99 98 97 96 95 94 93 92 91 90

10 9 8 7 6 5 4 3 2 1

Contents

–1–

The Winter of My Infertility

A MOUNTAIN ASH STOOD OUTSIDE MY BEDROOM WINDOW DURING the winter of my infertility. From time to time throughout that gray season, I looked up into its bare overhanging branches and prayed, "Just as spring will bring bud and blossom to this winter-blasted tree, so you, Lord, in your power can bring forth life in me." Winter slipped away, and with spring came white blossoms and bright orange berries to the once-barren tree, but spring did not come similarly to me. The child I prayed for was not to be.

When I was growing up, childlessness, like sex, was rarely mentioned. Scrupulous avoidance of the topic hinted there was something not only sad but a bit odd about childless couples. Yet I thought little about it.

Not until I went to college did I begin to be aware of the painful reality of childlessness. Through a biochemical quirk, a young psychology professor of mine had become infertile. (Actually, since her infertility was absolute, it would be technically correct to say that she was sterile.) Although only in her twenties, this strikingly beautiful woman had already gone through menopause. Firm in their desire for children, she and her husband sought to adopt as soon as her doctor's diagnosis was confirmed. Since they applied before the abortion legislation of the seventies and well before the current trend among single mothers to keep their babies, they waited only a few short months for a child. They were overjoyed when a hefty baby boy became theirs through adoption.

Later, when my husband and I were first married, we became acquainted with two couples in our church who had each been struggling to start a family. We sympathized with them, but we could not begin to grasp why they found their infertility so painful. As newlyweds anticipating several financially uncertain years of graduate school, we were unable to comprehend their sense of urgency. We were glad for the Pill!

Despite our contact with these couples, I still assumed that children were a given. You grew up, finished your education, got married, and had children. In due time, I hoped to have two of them myself—one boy and one girl—conveniently spaced two to three years apart. My expectations were as conventional as they were naive.

After we had been married for five years, my husband had nearly finished his doctorate, and I had completed a master's degree and was working. Our future looked more stable and predictable than it had when we first married, and we began to anticipate starting our family. We were then in our late twenties and aware that, from a strictly biological standpoint, our peak childbearing years were already past. Also, although there was no direct social pressure on us to have a child, we were beginning to find ourselves in the minority among our friends.

Couples in our church were having babies left and right, including our closest friends who had two small daughters. We gave those little girls lunch now and then, took them on outings to the neighborhood park, and were often part of their bedtime routine. A number of factors, including our almost daily association with that young family, combined to make us wish for a child of our own.

A doctor's incorrect diagnosis put an abrupt end to our hopes.

One fall weekend during my husband's last year of graduate school, I came down with an apparent case of flu. Although the symptoms were severe, I expected them to run their course quickly. Sunday afternoon, however, my temperature reached 105 degrees, and my husband insisted on taking me to the emergency room of the local hospital. There the physician on duty ordered a blood test and gave me a quick examination; he then prescribed some pills and sent me home, telling me that I had "the thing that's going around." Feeling rather foolish for going to the hospital for an apparently minor complaint, we accepted this diagnosis and went home.

About thirty-six hours later, I found myself in an ambulance and on my way back to the emergency room. By then my appendix had ruptured, and I had acute abdominal peritonitis. After immediate surgery, a stint in intensive care, and ten days of intravenous antibiotics, the infection was brought under control. Shortly after Thanksgiving I was discharged, and by Christmas I was beginning to feel like myself again. I had no inkling that my illness was to have lasting consequences.

As my strength returned that winter, my husband and I began to await the conception of a child expectantly. After several uneventful months, I became slightly concerned. Then I chanced upon a magazine article that enumerated several causes of infertility; one infrequent cause, mentioned merely in passing, was the side effects of a ruptured appendix. Ordinarily, infertility is not seriously suspected until twelve months of regular sexual relations have failed to result in conception. But that article sounded a small, persistent bell of warning in my mind and prompted me to consult a gynecologist without waiting any longer.

After putting me through an inconclusive round of preliminary tests and referring my husband to a urologist for a routine examination, my doctor recommended that I undergo an exploratory laparoscopy. A minor surgical procedure often used in tubal ligations performed on women who voluntarily surrender their fertility to surgery, a laparoscopy gives the physician a clear view of the abdominal cavity including the reproductive organs. Without delay, I was scheduled for surgery as an outpatient.

When I awoke from anesthesia on the morning of my laparoscopy and began to get my bearings, I noticed two nurses glancing from a chart to me and then back to the chart. From across the room I could lip-read a "That's too bad" from one nurse while the other nodded in mute agreement. "What's too bad?" I wondered. "Am I imagining things, or are they really talking about me?" Since they looked away when they caught me watching them, I had a sinking feeling that they were. But their attention was soon claimed by another patient. In an irony that others who are infertile will recognize as typical, the patient lying nearest me had just come from an abortion. She was hemorrhaging profusely, and her doctor, who was still in surgery, could not respond to the nurses' page. To complicate matters further, the frightened patient spoke only Spanish, and the nurses were unable to reassure her.

Into this confusion walked my doctor, looking too sober for my comfort. He helped me out of bed, sat me on a chair, and told me gently but firmly that my chances of having a child were slight at best. Infection resulting from my ruptured appendix had so scarred my Fallopian tubes that they were hopelessly blocked, even clubbed. The word "clubbed" shocked me, conjuring up disquieting images of disfigurement. Through a fog of anesthesia and faint nausea, I managed to ask whether micro-surgery, a relatively new technique full of promise for women with obstructed tubes, might possibly repair the damage. My doctor replied that scarring and adhesions were so extensive and the chances of success so minimal that he could not hold out that hope to me. Then he left, and a nurse led me to my clothes. The entire procedure had lasted little more than an hour, but in that time I felt like someone had cleanly and efficiently erased my expectations for the future.

More than ten years have passed since then, and I know now that specific responses to infertility are as individual and varied as those who experience it. However, there are several general themes that typically run through the experience of those who are involuntarily childless. Among these are surprise, a sense of isolation, diminished self-esteem, and confused self-image. In addition, once the initial feelings of disbelief and shock wear off, they are often replaced by anger and, in conclusive diagnoses, a profound sense of loss that can only be described as grief. The unthinking reactions of others and the strain of the infertility inves-tigation itself compound these feelings.

I can still recall how isolated I felt at first. My closest friend, a teacher, had timed the birth of her first child to coincide almost perfectly with the end of the school year. Her second child was also conceived on cue. Except for me, every woman in my weekly Bible study had at least one child. Even the farm animals in the surrounding countryside, whose young trailed bleating behind them, seemed to mock me.

I was soon surprised to discover, however, that I was hardly the rarity I had imagined. Barbara Eck Menning, founder of the Resolve organization and well-known infertility expert, estimates that at any given time some ten million Americans, or one of six couples of childbearing age, experience infertility.[1]

Furthermore, while single people tend not to be included in discussions of childlessness, it is a keenly felt issue for many who lack prospects of marriage and see the biological clock as operating against them.

In short, I have found that the involuntarily childless are a sizable minority. Within that minority are many Christians who are often struggling alone with their infertility, unaware that what they are experiencing is common to many others. Compounding the pain of infertility for Christians is the uneasy suspicion that since children are a sign of God's favor, their absence must be a sign of his judgment or displeasure. Complicating their struggle is the church, which is the most pro-natalist, or pro-birth, and pro-family of our institutions. A couple without children or an individual without a family can find the church a lonely, alienating place to be.

The following chapters, based on the stories of more than fifty infertile Christian couples from nineteen states, address a variety of infertility-related issues: the psychological and emotional aspects of infertility, the particular sorrow of miscarriage, the resolution of grief, and the decision whether to adopt or opt for "child-free" living. Although one chapter describes the infertility workup and surveys the causes and treatments of infertility, I have left it to those in the medical professions to comprehensively cover the physiological area. My primary concern is with exploring the emotional, psychological, social, and spiritual dimensions of this life crisis.

When I conducted my first interview for this book, the woman with whom I was talking challenged me by saying, "When I told my husband about this, he said, 'Is she going to interview any husbands too? It wasn't just you; it was me, too. We were in this together. This was our thing. Not yours. Not mine. But ours.'" Her husband is right, and most husbands, including mine, would agree.

Infertility is not primarily a female problem. There is a male problem in forty percent of infertility cases; in forty percent, there is a female problem; and in the remaining cases, there is a combination of difficulties. Regardless of where the medical cause lies, infertility is not the problem of the husband or the wife. It belongs to both, and both must pull together. While infertility is by no means merely a "women's issue," I have found that women express their feelings about infertility far more readily than men. I have also found that in the majority of cases women are more deeply affected by it. For these reasons, I have limited my interviews primarily to women, often trusting them to represent fairly their husband's point of view. There are, however, some special exceptions, and I am particularly indebted to those men who have contributed their experiences to this book.

In the course of conducting interviews and gathering research for this book, I was moved over and over again by the readiness of Christians to relate their experiences of infertility for the benefit of others. In a response characteristic of many, Margie, a thirty-one-year-old executive secretary from the Chicago area, said, "Thank you for allowing me to share in this way. It helps make the grief and pain of previous years worthwhile. I would love to think that God had used me in some small way in the lives of other childless women."

Margie's story together with those of Christian women and men from California to Florida appear in the following pages. They bear testimony to the fact that while we Christians are no more exempt from infertility than we are from the other struggles and challenges of human existence, we are never left alone and comfortless. If we let him, the Lord will walk with us through the narrow prisons of our disappointments and lead us into wider places. This is borne out repeatedly in the lives of those who have shared in this book. What often begins as songs of sorrow turns in time to songs of joy.

–2–

Infertility
*The Emotional
and Psychological Impact*

As MANY COUPLES ARE PAINFULLY AWARE, THE INFERTILITY INVEStigation itself is stressful. "Invasive" is the apt word often used to describe an infertility workup. Couples undergoing an infertility investigation typically find that sexual intercourse is programmed to coincide with the days of peak fertility and is therefore robbed of spontaneity. Having to "perform" according to the calendar or the reading on a basal thermometer does nothing to lessen the tension caused by infertility.

Tracy, an Oklahoma pastor's wife, recalls, "For the first time in our married life, sex became a chore for me instead of the blessed, uniting force it had been. I lost interest in making love on my nonfertile days because sex had become a purely procreative act. Sometimes I even cried during intercourse at the sheer futility of it all. During my supposedly fertile days, making a baby was my only goal. My husband was understanding and patient, but it couldn't have been easy for him either. Praise God, I've now progressed to the point where I can enjoy this gift of 'becoming one' again!"

In spite of their best efforts to stay cool and objective and tell themselves there is much to be gained, many women undergoing infertility tests feel violated. For example, when a woman undergoes a hysterosalpingogram, she lies with her feet in the cold steel stirrups of the gynecologist's table and watches, in the company of a doctor and an X-ray technician, while the pathway of dye injected into her uterus is monitored on a closed-circuit television screen. What is private becomes public. Finding oneself the subject of such clinical procedures is a shock, especially since they are far removed from all the warm pink-and-blue images we associate with having babies. Although infertility tests for women are more numerous than those for men, husbands do not escape them altogether. And it would be unusual if a man did not feel somewhat degraded and threatened by being asked to provide a semen sample so that his sperm might be evaluated.

Yet the infertility workup and the search for medical answers is only one dimension of infertility. As a couple spends hours waiting in their physician's outer offices, often in the company of hugely pregnant women, and faces the battery of tests one by one, the painful search for answers to difficult questions goes on: Why us? Where is God in all of this? Are we, for some mysterious reason, unworthy to be parents? Along with bewilderment and unfocused guilt come feelings of isolation, diminished self-esteem, anger, and grief. For Christians there is often a sense of being abandoned by God. The unthinking reactions of others frequently reinforce these feelings. As one California woman says, "When people in general become more informed about infertility, those suffering from it will have their trial divided in half."

Other's Reactions

Couples struggling with infertility must learn to handle the insensitive though well-intentioned advice of others. Particularly painful are the judgmental and spiritualizing comments that come from other Christians. The only thing that hurts more is when others avoid the issue altogether. The inherently sexual nature of infertility can cause others to shrink from discussing it, which leaves those who are infertile alone in their distress. A woman who eventually had two children recollects, "My husband and I became very close during our infertile years because we found so many friends and relatives to be unconscious of our grief." Another woman adds, "People think it's a 'shame' that we cannot have children, but no one seems to care how we *feel* about our infertility."

Unfortunately, when others do speak to the issue of infertility, their comments are often superficial or inappropriate. The most common misconception is that infertility is a psychological or spiritual problem rather than a medical condition.

Two toddlers play near their father, a young minister, who attempts to console an infertile couple by saying, "Don't worry. God may not have given you biological children, but he will give you spiritual children." Such platitudes may contain a grain of truth, but they too often gloss over a couple's legitimate grief and offer little or no comfort.

An earnest Christian couple who desperately want children are told by their fundamentalist parents that if they search out and find their sin, remove it from their lives, and exercise enough faith, they will conceive a child. To fail is to demonstrate a lack of faith. In this mechanistic theology, God is made a magician and prayer a magic formula, and Christianity becomes a means to manipulate God for what we want in life.

A California woman has heard a whole string of pat, sometimes contradictory pronouncements from her fellow Christians: "You're not praying enough." "Don't nag God with your prayers." "Be careful what you pray for. God may get tired of your prayers and give you a retarded child just to show you who's boss." "You don't have enough faith." "Your faith isn't pure enough."

The all-too-common insinuation that infertility is a consequence of sin and doubt, and fertility a reward for virtue and faith, is insupportable. There is simply too much evidence to the contrary. A recent Child Welfare League report, for example, gave a brief but shocking account of Kevin, a fourteen-month-old foster child who had been born to a thirteen-year-old mother; the mother is mildly retarded, emotionally disturbed, and presently in custody for delinquency. Kevin is a product of incest. Such tragic cases, which happen in one form or another every day, make a mockery of glib assertions about fertility and worthiness.

In coping with others' reactions, it is helpful to realize that people generally respond to infertility out of their own experience and circumstances. "Many people simply didn't know how to respond to us," recalls Joan. "For instance, my father-in-law's comment was, 'You're just as well off. I wouldn't want to have to raise a child in this day and age.' My sister said, 'Oh, you're so lucky not to have to worry about contraception.' At that time my father-in-law was going through some hard times with a teenaged daughter who had just had an abortion. My sister, on the other hand, had just married, and she wasn't at all interested in having children right off the bat. What it came down to was that people's comments were simply reflective of where they were."

In sorting out others' reactions, it is also helpful to understand that some Christians think they must have airtight answers to all of life's questions. Some of us are terribly uncomfortable with any ambiguity or mystery, and we cover our unease with pietistic slogans. On one hand, we claim to worship a God whose ways are too high for us and past finding out. On the other, we are at pains to explain him and his ways in great detail to ourselves and others.

Infertility is a sticky wicket for those whose theology does not allow for the possibility of unanswered questions. Leonard, trying very hard to come to terms with his sterility, sought the counsel of a minister. "When I told the minister about my zero sperm count," Leonard, says, "that seemed to catch him off guard. He asked if we'd tried any prayer and fasting! Prayer was the main thing we had been doing! He could only offer clichés. Our specific problem was too hard to handle."

Almost everyone who contributed to this book commented on the devastating impact of the uninformed and sometimes heartless comments of others. There are still times when my equilibrium is momentarily shaken by a tactless remark or blunt question, and to cope with the inevitable yet confounding probing of others, I have worked out some informal rules for myself.

1. In the case of simple bad manners, I rarely make a direct response, nor do I give in to the temptation to offer a quick course in childlessness. I let it go. And I try not to take offense. This is not always the best policy, however. Sometimes people need to be confronted with the effect of their words, not only for one's own sake but for the sake of the next person who might be wounded by their carelessness or ignorance.

One woman says, "My nice middle-class way is to say, 'Well, they don't know any better, so I'll just ignore it.' But sometimes those thoughtless comments or cutting remarks are too much, and I snap back. When I snap at someone, it's really an opportunity for them to become aware that we belong to each other and that their words do hurt. I don't think we ought always to suffer in silence. We ought to speak up when someone makes a thoughtless remark to us or other people who are not able to defend themselves. That's what I see Jesus doing a lot." I have gradually come to see that confronting someone with the impact of their words is both more honest and more honorable than pretending not to be hurt and seething with unspoken resentment or withdrawing in icy silence.

2. While I feel no need to explain our childlessness defensively to everyone, I make no secret of it. A simple word of explanation can head off awkwardness and misunderstanding. At a party my husband and I gave, a new acquaintance jokingly suggested that baby-sitting for his three active preschoolers would be excellent preparation for parenthood—an acid test of our patience. Knowing he meant well, I briefly explained that having children was not an option for us. He was thereby prevented from making more casual remarks that might later embarrass him.

Sometimes the best defense against misunderstanding is a good offense. A number of those with whom I have talked or corresponded have taken the positive step of seeking to inform their ministers and others close to them about infertility, and their efforts have frequently been rewarded. For example, a children's ministries director in a West Coast church says, "I have tried to 'educate' our ministers about infertility by talking with them and sharing a research paper I wrote for a graduate course in family and child development. I was delighted when our senior pastor made some sensitive remarks about infertility in his last Mother's Day sermon."

With family and others close to us, I am open about my infertility. I want my family and friends to know me, to understand me, and that, in part, depends on my being forthright about my childlessness. People cannot be held accountable for what they do not know. Furthermore, being open has helped me develop a healthy objectivity about my inability to have children. Being secretive only magnifies it out of proportion.

Yes, it is risky to be open about infertility; responses may well be disappointing. On the other hand, support often comes from unexpected quarters. My husband and I found that those who were the most helpful neither minimized nor exaggerated our loss. They permitted us to grieve but did not pity us.

Isolation

Leonard, a thirty-five-year-old Kansan, began his story with these poignant words: "While I *know* there must be other men like me, I don't *feel* like there are any others out there who are sterile and wish they could father their own kids." Complications arising from childhood surgery to correct an undescended testicle left Leonard with a zero sperm count. Since he knows no other infertile men, his sense of isolation is profound. Paradoxically, his condition is the envy of some of his male co-workers who wish they did not have to guard against unwanted pregnancies.

Many who are infertile feel alone and out of the social mainstream. A San Diego woman, who is now the mother of twin daughters, says, "When I was childless, I made the mistake of listening to people who said that parenting was more challenging and worthwhile than 'just' teaching school and being a wife. I felt shut out by a fertile world, unable to receive its acceptance until I had passed some sort of pregnancy-parenting challenge." Similarly, a woman with a long history of miscarriage, who is now the mother of an adopted daughter, says, "I had the impression that when friends talked about the birth process and childrearing, they were talking to me like I was a younger child. I was frustrated that I might never grow up and talk like the big kids."

For some, the conviction that they do not belong can find expression in furtive though innocent behavior. A woman from Wisconsin, who has experienced nine years of infertility, says, "Sometimes when I go shopping, I look through the infant clothes and other baby items. I feel guilty being in that department, sure that I will be spotted as an impostor and asked to leave the area." Another woman sheepishly admits to buying baby-care books and hiding them when guests come.

For others, infertility results in being bumped from an accustomed niche in one's family. Lynn, the eldest in a large midwestern family, says, "My great-grandmother, grandmother, mother, and myself have always enjoyed being four generations. Each year at mother-daughter banquets we get to stand. On one occasion, we had a four-generation portrait made. When my brother married several years after I did and then, in ten months, became a father, he and his wife and child took what was 'my' place in the portrait of five generations."

Such feelings of displacement hurt, and finding supportive others is an important step toward dealing with them. If God seems distant, a sympathetic touch, a listening ear, or the quiet understanding presence of another person can bring him nearer. Some couples plug into existing organizations; some build their own support systems. Often, finding just one understanding friend can make an enormous difference. "Nothing was as hurtful," states one woman, "as a friend who said, 'Hey, it's no big deal,' " and headed home with her toddler. Nothing was as helpful as a friend who said, 'I'm sorry this is happening to you.'" Although it is often most helpful to find others who share your struggle with infertility, it is certainly not essential. Two of the people who encouraged me most were a young mother of three who could practically conceive at will and a single professional woman to whom children were a dim, far-off concern.

A woman living in a small Eastern university town was feeling cut off from support and unsure where to turn. When she took the initiative to call the women's resource center at the university, she was given the name of another woman with an infertility problem. "I called her," she says, "and for the first time found someone I could sigh with, chat with, and cry with. She understood. What grew out of our conversation was the start of an infertility support group. We began to discover that there were a number of people in the community who needed to be together and talk. In addition to discussing our problems, we pooled information about the best doctors, clinics, and adoption agencies. In a few years, we grew from a group of five to thirty."

A Michigan woman has found strength in a far-flung group of correspondents. "For over four years," she says, "I had no one to share with. Now, miraculously, the Lord has given me a network of pen pals who have all experienced infertility and who now have babies by birth or adoption. I'm so grateful for these women who don't criticize but who understand and pray. People are often unwilling to pray right to the issue of infertility. As one of my friends says, 'Why do others always pray for peace for me? Why can't they pray for a baby?' That's a legitimate prayer, and the ones who have said, 'I will pray,' have been very encouraging."

Two organizations that offer resources to infertile couples and can help them make connections with others are Stepping Stones and Resolve. Stepping Stones is a nonprofit Christian ministry founded in 1981 by Lynn Campbell Behnke, Leslie Snodgrass, and Janet Malcom "to offer hope, encouragement, and support to infertile couples." The three founders form the Stepping Stones editorial board, and they publish a newsletter every two months, which is available free on request. Stepping Stones, which operates under the auspices of the Central Christian Church of Wichita, Kansas, is a lifeline for thousands of childless Christians.

Resolve, a secular organization much larger than Stepping Stones, was founded by Barbara Eck Menning. The services offered by this national, nonprofit organization (based in the Boston area) include telephone counseling, referrals to the best medical care and professional counseling, a network of support groups, and excellent literature, including the *Resolve* newsletter, which is available for a modest membership fee. (See appendix for addresses.)

Diminished Self-Esteem

Often reinforcing the isolation felt by infertile persons is a loss of self-esteem. For centuries, barrenness has been perceived as a disgrace, and, even today, in some cultures, it is regarded as sufficient grounds for divorce. While many still feel the stigma of infertility, not all infertile men and women find their self-esteem diminished. Margaret, for example, did not. A plain-spoken New Englander, she says, "I never felt less of a woman. I just felt a void. I wanted to have a child not to prove myself as a woman but to meet a need to have someone to care for, someone to take the overflow of our love." Like Margaret, some men do not feel diminished by their infertility. Commenting on her husband's reaction to his sterility, a Pennsylvania woman says, "I was surprised by how well he handled it. Male friends of ours said they would have been shattered. He simply accepted it."

Increasing social acceptance of childlessness and rapid changes in women's roles have reduced some of the stigma of being without child today. Still, the self-confidence of many is undermined by infertility. Tracy recalls, "My husband was relieved to learn that his sperm count was within the normal range, but that news caused me to view myself as the villain in this drama of infertility. I hated myself at times, especially during my periods. My inability to conceive became the focal point of my existence; it was all I thought about. I felt like an incomplete woman, a prepubescent freak, barely even a human being." A Tennessee woman adds, "I felt like a failure. Because our parents wanted to be grandparents and had no grandchildren, I felt like I was letting everyone, especially myself, down."

Infertile men as well as infertile women often find their self-esteem threatened. Leonard, who was in the Air Force during his first infertility workup, heard about his sterility from a lab technician who mistakenly assumed he had undergone a vasectomy. "Congratulations!" the technician said, "No sperm seen."

"I'd always been so cool," Leonard recalls, "thinking I was doing all this medical stuff for my wife. I began to realize I was also doing it for me. I sat and stared dumbly straight ahead and discovered there was a whole lot more sorrow inside than I had known. It shook me to the core."

Dan, a Florida high-school teacher and football coach, remembers, "I was numb with shock at first, and then I began to feel that God had cursed me. Because I could not father a child, I also began to feel less than a man. Despite the fact that my parents and my wife's parents and everyone we told were very reassuring, the feeling that I was inadequate, that there was something wrong with me, stuck in my mind."

Critical to the self-image of an infertile person is the support of his or her spouse. It is difficult to exaggerate the importance of communication and mutual support. As Dan says, "The problem of childlessness never strikes just one person or the other; it always strikes the couple. It's crucial that partners reach out to each other."

We are given to each other in marriage for keeps, for better or for worse, and whose "fault" infertility is should be of no real consequence. When the cause of a couple's infertility can be traced to one partner, however, fear of rejection often follows. As a midwesterner admits, "My husband's former girl friends have all had children, and I thought he might wish he had married one of them. The infertility problem was mine, and I was afraid he had regrets about marrying me. I carried that for a very long time before I had the courage to ask him if that was how he felt." Such fears are common and cannot be easily or quickly erased. Dispelling them requires patient reassurance and repeated affirmation.

It is also important to a healthy self-image to understand that infertility does not cancel out sexuality. There is more to sexuality than reproduction. A man, though his sperm count is zero, remains a man. A woman, though her chances of bearing a child are ever so slim, remains a woman. In the vast majority of cases, infertility has *nothing* to do with sexual inadequacy.

Another step toward a sound self-image is to resist accepting the term "infertile" as a definition of who you are. Some involuntarily childless people insist on hanging that label on themselves like a leper's bell. "Infertile" is a *descriptive* rather than a *definitive* term and might be one of hundreds of adjectives that could be applied to you; it does not begin to tell your whole story. For example, while vocation and participation in volunteer ministries do not take the place of children, they can be significant sources of identity and self-esteem.

Some turn their infertility into an opportunity for sharpening their vocational focus or investing more time in other people's lives. Tracy says, "I'm more confident in my teaching ability now. Being childless gave me the time and impetus to become the best teacher I could possibly be, and I feel that, with the Lord's help, I've succeeded in that area. At the time I was in the deepest sorrow over my infertility I was also trying to adjust to being a minister's wife, since my husband and I had just completed theological seminary and had moved to a full-time pastorate. Trying to be a 'smilingly spiritual saint' yet hating myself inside was very difficult.

"Gradually, I learned to be myself as a minister's wife, to draw fulfillment from my teaching career, and to be open with others about my infertility. I now feel that I am a valuable person—to God, my husband, the church, my fellow educators, and my schoolchildren. Even though I don't have a working set of reproductive organs, that makes me no less a Christian than someone who has five children. My husband was very good about constantly reassuring me concerning my womanhood, so I now feel like a complete woman once again, too."

Many childless Christians find that involvement in volunteer ministry, like vocational involvement, lends meaning to the present. Margie and her husband, Ray, are a Chicago-area couple who love children. They have found they can have an impact on them without being parents. "Last year," says Margie, "my husband became the Christian-education director of a Korean church. While this has taken up a lot of our spare time, it has been very rewarding. We both enjoy working cross-culturally, and the parents of these children appreciate our involvement too. While the parents are first-generation Americans, the children are very Americanized; to some extent, we're mediators between the generations. Exposure to these Korean children has made us interested in foreign adoption, and just being with them revitalizes me and gives me hope for the future."

Involvement in the present need not always take the form of service or of working with children. Many who wish to be parents are not particularly drawn to other people's children, and there are many worthwhile activities that do not fall neatly into the category of ministry. Perhaps, for example, you could get on with learning to play the piano. Perhaps you could develop your interest in watercolors, gardening, Chinese history, weaving, dancing, Dutch painting, or refinishing old pieces of furniture. Pursuing such interests is helpful in breaking up self-absorption and developing God-given capacities.

One of the outlets my husband and I have found for our energy and creativity is renovating the two old houses we have owned. It is satisfying to bring dull wood floors back to life, to patch aging plaster and brighten it with fresh paint, to turn cramped, dark spaces into light, inviting rooms. Our house feels grateful for our efforts, all of which contribute to making a home, if not for children, then for ourselves and all those with whom we share our lives. Such involvement in the present is important, since, as Margie says and as many childless people are keenly aware, "It's the not knowing from month to month that gets to you. If you could know that in five years you would conceive and have a child, you could get on with your life; but you simply can't live your life solely in anticipation of the future."

Guilt

A poor self-image and guilt feelings often go hand-in-hand. One infertile friend, plagued by a consistently low estimate of herself, says, "I feel like 'fate' has pointed a finger at me, saying I don't deserve to be pregnant, that I'm not good enough to be a mother."

This woman's fear that her infertility is a punishment for some un-defined inadequacy or sin is commonplace. In fact, as the following example illustrates, some couples fear being misunderstood and censured for things they have not even done: "We are Catholics. Not a week goes by that I don't hear that familiar portion of the Mass asking us to add our intentions to the prayer. Every week I ask God to grant us a child. I light vigil candles. I pray to Mary. Surely as a mother she will understand and intercede for me. I am afraid that priests and fellow parishioners who do not know me and our situation will assume that we do not follow the teachings of the Church and that we practice birth control. What else can you assume about a young healthy couple married nine years with no children! Once, when I was in confession, I confessed to the sin of being jealous toward a friend because she was pregnant, while I could not conceive a child. Mostly, I confessed this sin because it was true, but I also confessed it because I wanted the priest to know that I was an infertile Catholic, not a bad Catholic."

Given the sexual overtones of infertility, it is not surprising that guilt feelings often arise from sexual behavior, even when it is innocent. Common sources of guilt among the infertile not only include premarital and extramarital sex, abortion, and venereal disease but also the use of birth control and even sexual pleasure itself. Rarely, however, is there a rational basis for self-recrimination. We have about as much control over our fertility as we have over the color of our eyes or the size of our feet. And if children were a reward for virtue, and barrenness a punishment for sin—if it were really that simple— then fewer scoundrels and more saints would be having them.

Consider the case of Zechariah and Elizabeth, the parents of John the Baptist. They are described in Luke's gospel as "upright in the sight of God, observing all the Lord's commandments and regulations blamelessly. "But," Luke adds, "they had no children, because Elizabeth was barren; and they were both well along in years" (Luke 1:6-7).

Later, after the angel announced John's coming to Zechariah and Elizabeth was carrying him, she said, "The Lord has done this for me . . . In these days he has shown his favor and taken away my disgrace among the people" (Luke 1:25). Where was her disgrace? *Among the people.* Here the stigma of infertility is clearly social and has absolutely nothing to do with the judgment of God upon her life.

Of course our actions are not without consequences, and if an infection from an abortion has left us infertile, that is a fact with which we must live. Though our remorse may be great, the scarring and adhesions remain. Yet I would be very careful about trying to establish cause-and-effect relationships between past behavior and present infertility. If, for instance, there really was a one-to-one correspondence between sexual impurity and infertility, I think we would see a drop in the birthrate that would make our heads spin.

When guilt is not based merely on vague feelings but rooted in sin, the only recourse is to pray:

Have mercy on me, O God,
   according to your unfailing love;
according to your great compassion
   blot out my transgressions.
Wash away all my iniquity
   and cleanse me from my sin.   *Psalm 51:1-2*

Because it sometimes gives us the illusion of atoning for our misdeeds, we would rather hug our guilt to ourselves and wallow in the bog of self-abasement than accept the forgiveness offered us.

Remember when Jesus was with the woman caught in adultery? First he silenced her accusers by reminding them that none are guiltless. Then, turning to her and asking what had become of those who were about to stone her, he said, "Neither do I condemn you. Go and sin no more." Although it might have taken her some time to forget her shame and forgive herself, Jesus had forgiven her from that moment on, and he urged her to "Go"—to get on with her life rather than remain prostrate with remorse.

I know that letting go of guilt is often easier said than done. We may be well versed in the Scriptures and able to reel off such verses as "For as high as the heavens are above the earth, so great is his love for those who fear him; as far as the east is from the west, so far has he removed our transgressions from us" (Psalm 103:11-12). We may know that our sins are forgiven through the atoning death of Jesus Christ—that "nothing in our hands we bring, simply to his cross we cling." Yet we may still be plagued with crippling guilt feelings. With tears in her eyes, a minister's daughter says, "I have some guilt I'm having a hard time dealing with. I try to be rational about it. I read the Scripture passages, and I try to lay my life out in front of God, but I can't get rid of it." In such cases, seeking out a Christian counselor is recommended. The Lord has given us to each other, and he often uses our fellow Christians, including trained therapists and pastoral counselors, to help free us and bring his love and truth home to us.

In the following account, Anne, a professional artist, tells how other Christians helped her make the journey from guilt and self-hate to the freeing realization of God's forgiveness and unconditional love. "Two months after we were married," Anne says, "we realized we were over thirty, and we realized also that ours was not just a half-hearted commitment. We were going to stick it out regardless. We knew that there would be rocky times in our fiftieth year as well as our first year of marriage. So after being on the Pill for only two months, we began trying to start a family. We thought we would get pregnant immediately.

"When I didn't get pregnant that first month, or the second, or the third, I began to hear an inner voice that said, 'Well, of course. You're never going to be a mother. You're not good enough.' I've always had a poor self-image. This wasn't a voice that just started speaking to me when I got married and we started trying to have children. It didn't start even a few years before that. It's a voice that I think has always been with me. It's almost like another person."

Anne's chronically low self-image was reinforced by guilt over premarital sex. Yet she notes, "Whether my sexual behavior or my behavior in general had been near perfection or near the gutter, self-image would still have been a problem." She was always striving to meet standards that eluded her. Her sense of never quite measuring up resulted in part from her parents' expectations. She says, "I can remember watching a beauty pageant on television as a child and hearing my father say, 'Someday you're going to be in that pageant.' Then, when my brothers didn't go to college, Father put all of his hopes on me. I was the one who had to make the honor society and get the A's. On my mother's side, there was the expectation that my marriage at its worst would at least be as good as hers."

Even though the cause of their infertility had not been diagnosed, Anne assumed it must be her fault rather than her husband's. Infertility, she believed, was just one more confirmation of her inadequacy, one more hurdle she couldn't quite clear. As the infertility investigation continued without yielding any answers, she began to withdraw into herself. She felt alone in her church with its exploding baby population and remembers thinking, "If nothing else, it's got to be contagious! It seemed everybody was pregnant."

"We stopped the infertility testing, and although our infertility hadn't been resolved, I thought I was going to go on with my life. Instead, this veil came over me. I felt hopeless. I thought, 'Nobody understands,' and I can remember thinking, 'God is so far from me.' I'd given up on knowing that sense of security, that feeling of being in God's care. But I didn't blame him; I blamed myself."

During this trying time, Anne was suddenly hospitalized for a slightly perforated colon. That seemingly unfortunate event became a turning point. "When I went into the hospital," she says, "people started sending cards and flowers and coming to see me. When I came home from the hospital, the church started bringing dinners just like they do for new mothers! It began to dawn on me, 'People care. People really love me.' I was overwhelmed by their kindness.

"My pastor also helped. I was trying to make sense of my infertility, to make it fit theologically. I had been taking seminary classes, and for one of my courses I had even written a paper titled, 'The Childless Couple in God's Plan.' I shared the paper with my pastor who read it carefully and responded, 'I really can't believe that infertility is in God's plan any more than mental retardation is.' He helped me begin to see my infertility as a consequence of living in a fallen world rather than a curse that God had put on me because of my unworthiness.

"During this time, God's love came home to me not through a lightning bolt, not through any Scripture jumping out at me, but through his people—the only way I was ever going to see it. That was such a turning point, such a beautiful turning point, in my life.

"I came home from the hospital and continued to heal physically and spiritually. The more I thought about how I had come to a renewed awareness of God's love for me, the more I wanted to extend that love.

For the first time, adoption began to be an attractive alternative rather than merely an out. Before, I had said, 'God loves me but knows I wouldn't be a good mother.' Now I realized how absurd that was. I realized there are no 'buts' to God's love. I saw that he not only loved me but loved what I had the potential to become, and I began to affirm that I had the capacity to be a good mother. I have a whole new outlook that started, and had to start, with a clearer understanding of the unconditional nature of his acceptance. Now there's a bright sky instead of a dark tunnel."

Anger

Like feelings of isolation, low self-esteem, and guilt, anger is also a common response to infertility. Sometimes it is rational and has an object; sometimes it is the unfocused result of frustration. Anger has many faces:

"This is an angry period of time. A pessimistic period. I traveled home to remember the anniversary of my grandfather's death. I had wanted him to know the joy of a great-grandchild."

"A close relative told me, 'You're a Christian. You should be over this miscarriage by now.' I think my mouth must have dropped open a foot. How dare this woman who has never gone through any problems with pregnancy say something like that to me? She's never experienced what it's like to lose a life and go through all that anguish. I was absolutely furious."

"I got to the point of not turning the news on. It seemed like every single night I'd hear about a child-abuse case or the abortion issue. It was tearing me apart."

"My blocked tubes resulted from an IUD-related infection. In retrospect, I feel the infertility specialist should have suspected such a problem, but I am even more disturbed by the lack of communication on the part of the doctor who gave me the IUD in the first place."

"I remember my mother-in-law patting my stomach and asking, 'Is there anything in there for *me* yet?' Once, after tolerating that a number of times, I went to the bathroom, slammed the door, and stayed in there for a long time. She never said anything like that again."

"One evening I marched into the kitchen where my husband was sitting and said, 'I'm going to the doctor to get inseminated!' He got a hurt look on his face and said he didn't think he could handle it. We talked about it for hours, and I finally said, 'Well, how do you think I feel? I want to have your baby. That's my real desire, and I'm just frustrated. I don't think I could actually go through with artificial insemination.' We ended up by crying and holding each other."

As these examples illustrate, anger has various objects—abortion advocates, those who neglect or abuse their children, doctors, one's spouse. In addition, many who are infertile feel angry with and betrayed by God. One woman dealt constructively with her anger at God by writing him "letters." She says, "It helps me to write a letter to the Lord and pour out my heart to him. If I felt like he was being unfair, I told him so. If I was mad at him, I'd tell him and say, 'Lord, I don't understand this!' Sometimes I hurt so badly that words wouldn't come when I tried to pray, but I could write them down. It's interesting now to look back and see the spiritual growth that has occurred." Her practice of keeping an honest record of an intimate relationship with the Lord has a parallel in the Psalms. David, "a man after his (God's) own heart" (1 Samuel 13:14), not only offers worship and praise to God in the Psalms, he also blasts God for his apparent absence and seeming forgetfulness of his promises.

Anger often flares up within marriage when infertility becomes an issue. Since infertility carries sufficient pain within itself, it is most unfortunate when that pain is compounded by marital strife. But blaming and being angry at one's spouse are not at all unusual. However irrational it may be, such hostility should be owned and resolved rather than buried. It can be long indulged only at the risk of the relationship. If feelings are too hot to handle and you fear doing irreparable harm to your marriage, seek out a mediator—a minister or marriage counselor or an especially wise and trusted friend. Although getting potentially explosive feelings out in the light can be risky, it is considerably safer than nurturing them in silence where they can grow out of all reasonable proportion.

The need for openness, particularly within marriage, is underscored by Joan, who says, "It's important to allow each other to voice feelings. I remember a tender moment during the week we found out we couldn't bear children when Bill found me upstairs crying my eyes out. He hugged me and we cried together. That was very special. It's also important to allow the stages of the hurt to happen, to let them surface rather than repress them. They will come out in one way or another, and it does no good to bury them. Obviously, the end result is to arrive at a pretty healthy state."

While it may be directed at one's spouse or another specific object, anger often arises not from a single cause but from the piling up of losses and indignities. A nurse with a long, painful medical history, including multiple miscarriages and a precancerous condition that led to a total hysterectomy, says, "Even though I am a member of the medical profession, I have a lot of anger. There was the cold, calculating marking of an X on the temperature chart each time we had intercourse. There was the lack of privacy as everyone watched an 'interesting hysterosalpingogram.' After surgery, I woke up alone, grieving on cold stretchers. That 'rotten uterus' was useless to me, and yet what a loss I felt after the hysterectomy. At first I was extremely angry about those losses. It was not only the lack of children. It was that a whole chunk of my life and marriage had been given to this. And for this huge investment there was not much payoff. Bitterness is my concern. How do I resolve these issues so they do not end in bitterness?"

Perhaps the best answer to this difficult question is that Jesus feels the pain beneath the surface of our anger. He understands the hurt underlying our bitterness, and he wants to touch and heal us. Marjory Bankson, the president of Faith at Work, has some pertinent observations on this subject. Speaking about the ministry of Jesus to "bent women," Marjory says, "A story that touches me every time I read it is the story of the bent woman (Luke 13:10-17). It's only a few verses long and takes place on a Sabbath. Jesus apparently goes from the men's side of the synagogue over to the women's side because he is moved with compassion for this woman who is bent over. And he heals her; he straightens her up. That's all we see of the woman. Then the Pharisees take him to task for healing on the Sabbath.

"That is a rather poignant story for me. What it says to me is that Jesus was aware of the bent women around him and certainly much more aware of the plight of women than his disciples were. Think of all the interactions he had with women: the woman who was healed of the issue of blood; the woman at the well about whom the disciples could only say, 'Why is he talking to that woman?'; the prostitute who came to Simon's house and washed his feet with her hair only to hear, 'Well, if he only knew who was touching him, he wouldn't allow that.'

"Jesus seemed to be particularly aware of women and their needs as well as their capacities for love. As far as I can tell, none of these women were mothers. They were all women whom Jesus called to a kind of strength and even missionary role. That is, he called them to bear witness to what he had done in their lives.

"Jesus calls us first of all to be healed. That does not necessarily mean infertility will vanish or that all the scars will be erased. Yet whether or not the infertility itself is healed, he calls us to be healed of those emotions that have plagued and crippled us. And then he calls us to move on with our lives and bear witness to that healing."

There is healing in Christ for the hurts of infertility, and that is good news indeed. As we shall see in the next chapter, however, the road to healing is sometimes long and circuitous.

–3–

When Grief Fails

WHEN INFERTILITY IS ABSOLUTE, OR WHEN A COUPLE GIVES UP ON biological children after years of unsuccessful treatment and disappointed hopes, grief usually follows. Although it is a mistake to try to forestall grief, many attempt to avoid it through losing themselves in their work or by immediately launching into adoption proceedings. Some take refuge in overspending or overeating. Others find themselves strangely listless and apathetic and retreat into television or escapist fiction.

One infertile Christian couple unconsciously tried to postpone their grieving by taking elaborate trips and going on shopping sprees. They caught themselves, quit trying to fill the void in their lives by artificial means, and allowed themselves to grieve. Only then were they able to see their options clearly and determine what was most important to them. They found that grieving, though painful, was a necessary step in the resolution of their infertility. This was certainly true in my own experience as well.

It was the Friday morning of my laparoscopy. With obvious reluctance, my doctor had just told me that in all probability I would never bear children. I listened stonily to his description of the extent of the damage resulting from my ruptured appendix. I asked several short questions, and I willed a quick end to our conversation. There was nothing in his guarded manner or in the atmosphere of the recovery room to encourage any show of feeling on my part. Lit up as brightly as a highway rest stop and full of strangers, that room seemed an inhospitable place from which I could not escape fast enough. I wanted my husband and the comfort and safety of his presence.

Dick and I made the twenty-minute drive from the hospital to our house in silence, tacitly agreeing to hold off all talk until we were home. We were both numb. We spent the day quietly, he working at his desk, me sleeping off the after-effects of the anesthesia. We had been invited to have dinner with our closest friends that evening and watch the television debut of a young actress whom we all knew. We kept the engagement because we did not want to be alone, and we could depend on our friends for an easy, companionable evening. They and their children were like family to us during our graduate-school years in Pennsylvania.

Our friends had worked hard that day, shopping for and preparing a special lobster dinner, little thinking that the outcome of my laparoscopy would be so bleak. Oddly enough, the last occasion on which the four of us had thrown a lobster dinner had also turned out quite inauspiciously. For me, lobster was fast becoming a curious emblem of disaster. After dinner, with me tucked under a quilt on their sofa, we settled in to watch the television show. It was a standard hospital drama, and none of us were nearly as interested in the plot as we were in the performance of our actress friend.

Five minutes into the program, we discovered that she was cast as an unwed mother. There wasn't anything to do but laugh. The evening brought a fictional example of an undesired pregnancy. That morning I had awakened from anesthesia a few beds away from an abortion patient. On the day when my infertility was sealed, there were signs of unwanted fecundity on every hand. We made an early night of it.

By the next morning, the shock that had insulated us for the first twenty-four hours or so and given us a bit of breathing room had worn off. Grief hit with an almost physical force, stunning us both. We had known that if we discovered we could not have children, it would hurt; neither of us had realized how much. In the midst of our private, individual sorrow, we were given the grace to cling tightly to each other. There was no thought of recrimination, of drawing apart. Instead, we groped blindly for each other, seeking and finding wordless solace.

That weekend I felt engulfed by despair, by a mental blackness that was frightening in its intensity. As I went about the house performing simple tasks, it was as though I were drowning, pushed to the bottom of a dark pool and held there by an unseen hand. Anything resembling formal prayer was beyond me. Yet at the worst moments, I was given the grace to call silently on the name of Christ, saying within myself simply, "Jesus, Jesus." And help came. The waters receded. I could breathe. The awful weight of darkness lifted momentarily until the next wave hit. Again I would silently call, "Jesus." As quickly as he was there for the man called Peter who slipped, terrified, into the sea, he was there for me.

During that weekend we allowed ourselves to touch bottom, to let grief wash over us. We did so not out of masochism or a taste for melodrama but out of a partly subconscious realization that it was the only way to get to the other side of the pain. Had we fully understood what we were letting ourselves in for, we may have found ways to evade or at least postpone our grieving. By Monday morning, however, the worst was over. The storm had broken. Grief would, of course, recur and take some time to resolve, but it would never recur to the same paralyzing extent.

Before my infertility I had already learned what grief feels like. In the first years of our marriage, my two younger brothers died within six months of each other. They were barely into their twenties, and only eleven months separated me from my nearest brother, Robby, with whom I was especially close. The pain of losing them, like the pain of childlessness, drove my husband and me together and taught us some early lessons in grieving. Apart from those experiences, I am not sure that we would have understood so quickly that the only way to deal with any grief, including the sorrow of infertility, is to walk through it. There is simply no going around it. If denied, it will simply resurface months or even years later.

When Dick and I discovered our infertility, we had the somewhat dubious advantage of having already learned what it is to mourn. What of the many young couples for whom infertility is the first serious life crisis they must face? How do they interpret their experience? What context, I wonder, do they have for their sorrow? It is not surprising that the most common problem Barbara Eck Menning has encountered in her years of counseling infertile clients is the failure or inability to grieve.

According to Menning, one of the primary reasons for failed grief is that there may be no recognized loss. She notes that since the grief of infertility is over the loss of potential life rather than actual life, a couple may not realize they are entitled to grieve.[1] The nebulousness of this grief can interfere with its resolution. There is no face, no set of memories attached to it. There is no funeral and none of the other rituals that accompany death in our society to mark it off as a time of mourning. Instead, there is the death of dreams and the end, perhaps, of a family name. One woman has described it as grief for all of the children she will never have.

The Cost of Silence

Even when there is a recognized loss, isolation can occur for a couple unable to share the pain of their infertility with others. Unfortunately, silence serves only to short-circuit grief. Tracy, the pastor's wife quoted at the beginning of the second chapter, has firsthand experience of trying to go it alone. "As our friends, couple by couple, achieved the fulfillment of their dreams and became pregnant, I withdrew further and further into myself. Each baby shower was torture—selecting a gift to be used by someone else's baby, listening to conversations about breastfeeding, and trying to put on a cheerful front through it all. My friends would say, 'Well, Tracy, you'll be next!' Instead of being honest and saying, 'I sure hope so,' I developed an unhealthy habit of trying to deceive even my closest friends.

"I lied to many people and told them that after a long talk, Les and I had reached the conclusion our careers were more important to us than having a family at this stage of our lives. I even said I had gone back on the Pill, pretending it was my *choice* not to be pregnant. Meanwhile I cried in private, felt terribly guilty about my falsehoods, and we continued our feverish quest for conception. For nearly two years we told no one, family or friends, what we were going through.

"Well-meaning church people would sometimes ask us when we were going to start a family. We'd make our usual round of excuses, and I'd be close to tears. People would tell us we needed to 'fill up' the guest rooms in the parsonage, and I'd force myself to laugh at their well-intentioned humor, again making excuses. I feared people would reject me if they knew my 'shameful secret.'

"My turning point came when, thank God, I started opening up and sharing my feelings of frustration with Christian friends closest to me. First I wrote letters to several friends and relatives in other places. Their loving support gave me the courage to share my private grief with a very special local friend, a member of our church. She has an adopted daughter, has experienced the agony of several miscarriages, and could truly understand my pain. In this one friend I found a wellspring of empathy and encouragement. Every infertile woman should know someone like Linda!

"I then began opening up to other people, both teacher-friends and church friends. Honesty and openness freed me tremendously, but I did learn to be careful about the people with whom I shared some things. Even Christians who haven't been there sometimes have trouble understanding the grief that goes along with infertility. For example, several of our friends were critical of my decision not to attend a church mother-daughter banquet. But the majority of the people with whom I shared the trauma of infertility showed love and support even though they didn't always understand my exact feelings. As one special teacher-friend put it, 'I can't always precisely relate to your experiences, but since I love you as a sister in Christ, I can feel your pain somewhat, cry with you, and help you bear this burden.'

"At the urging of my minister-husband, I also began seeing a Christian pastoral counselor for help in coping with infertility. My counselor listened to me vent feelings of anger, grief, and fear, and she helped me deal with them. She even cried with me on occasion! As a result of our weekly sessions, I began feeling much more relaxed and in tune with the

Lord. She also helped me understand that God grieves with us and offers us a limitless reservoir of comfort and compassion when we face life's rough spots."

Finding Supportive Others

In beginning to open up about her infertility, Tracy found help; she began to develop a support system that sustained her, and she began to deal constructively with her infertility. The critical role that supportive others can play in the resolution of grief is further illustrated by the experience of Dan, a Florida teacher, and his wife, Kathy.

During a vacation visit with family in Michigan, Kathy and Dan arranged to see an infertility specialist. Their problem was quickly diagnosed: Dan was irreversibly sterile. "I was fully prepared when we went to the doctor's office to hear that Kathy was having problems with being fertile," Dan acknowledges. "I never in a million years expected the doctor to say that I was sterile. The news drastically affected our marriage. The communication gap was instant. Whenever I have a problem, I tend to internalize my feelings. This thing seemed intensely personal to me, and it was nothing I thought Kathy could share."

Kathy recalls, "I was more angry at the news than anything else. I felt it was God's fault for putting some sort of curse on us. I was angry at him, angry at my husband, and angry at myself. At the same time, we also desired to comfort one another, but we didn't know how. We didn't know what words to say. We were stunned into silence."

Since they were visiting family when the news of Dan's sterility came, Kathy and Dan initially received the warm and loving support of their parents and friends. When their visit ended, however, they returned to their jobs in Florida and to a house that suddenly seemed terribly empty. Having lived in Florida for only a year, they were still in the process of deciding on a church and making new friends. They felt alone, and their silence and estrangement from each other grew. Convinced that the silence would soon destroy their marriage, they began making plans to return to Michigan where they could be among family and friends.

While they were in the midst of planning their move, a family from the church they had been visiting invited them to come for Thanksgiving dinner. That simple gesture proved to be a gift of grace. "We walked in the door," Kathy says, "and we felt a load had been lifted from us even though nothing had been said. The family was very warm and caring, much like the one in which I grew up. People were constantly coming and going. We literally lost ourselves in the life that was present in that home.

"In the days that followed, we were often together, talking for hours at a stretch and getting to know one another. We were soon able to open up and tell them that we were having a problem coping with our childlessness. They also began to share their life with us, and we learned that they had lost their first child and that loss had put a considerable strain on their marriage. Because we could see they had survived a difficult time, they offered hope to us. They were also safe people with whom we could release the emotions of shock, disbelief, and anger that had been dammed up. They provided a buffer zone, and we could safely let everything out to them. Finally, healing could begin. Christ was present to us in them."

Although there are still times when they withdraw out of fear of rejection or when they are tempted to strike out at each other, Dan and Kathy have been learning to talk about their infertility. The gradual healing of their relationship continues. They have dropped their plans to move, and they have made considerable progress toward adoption. Through the loving intervention of fellow Christians, the silence that could have cost them their marriage has lifted.

The Need for Inner Healing

When grief fails for a prolonged period, the cost can be terribly high. Holly and David suffered for five long years. Before I met Holly, a friend of hers said, "Holly has been away for a long time. Now she's back." Only after hearing Holly's story did I begin to understand that enigmatic remark.

One spring morning, after not feeling well for several weeks, Holly awoke with abdominal pain too persistent to ignore. She stayed home from work, and finally, after she had recovered from blacking out in the bathroom, she called David. By the time they reached the hospital later that day, her pain was so severe that the examining physician had to give her Demerol before he could touch her. The doctor quickly diagnosed an ectopic or tubal pregnancy, which had probably already ruptured the tube in which it was implanted. Holly was prepared for immediate surgery to remove the tube that had burst.

In addition to being a medical emergency, an ectopic pregnancy usually comes as a complete surprise, and a woman's emotional reaction is often delayed. Unaware that she has conceived, she is bewildered by the sudden loss of a pregnancy she never knew she had. This was true in Holly's case. "Although the doctor explained to me what had happened," she recalls, "it did not sink in until later." Raised with a belief in a God who was primarily a God of judgment rather than love, Holly later felt guilty, angry, and depressed. She says, "My mother had always said, 'Don't ever go on the Pill. That's tampering with God's territory.' Early in our marriage I was on the Pill for nine months before I decided to go off because of possible side effects. When I had the ectopic pregnancy, I thought, 'See, God's punishing me because I was on the Pill for nine lousy months. He's getting revenge.' I know that is really stupid now, but that's how I felt at the time."

Adding to the emotional and physical strain of Holly's pregnancy was a succession of trying events, including an ovarian cyst and a lump on one breast. In addition, her father began to have heart trouble. "All of this was piling up inside me," she admits, "and I wasn't dealing with it. I had never experienced anything I couldn't handle on my own, but I didn't know how to cope with all of this. I was angry at God without realizing at first that I was, and I took my anger out mainly on David. Constant criticism. Constant nagging. He couldn't do a single thing right, no matter how hard he tried. I've since learned that there is nothing wrong with expressing anger to God. But at the time I thought, 'How could I do that? I'll never get to heaven!'

"Through the past five years I've been in varying states of depression. I've had periodic up times, but most of the time I have been in severe depression. During this time, I couldn't even see the beauty in a flower or in any aspect of God's creation. I didn't want to cook. I wouldn't clean. I didn't want to go out anywhere. I didn't want to have people in. David would suggest something, and I would say, 'No, I'm too tired.' If I had been married to anyone less sympathetic and understanding, we would probably be divorced at this point. I really put him through hell. He would come home from work after a long day and find no dinner and the house in a mess. He'd not only go about making dinner, but he'd do the dishes afterward. This went on for years.

"Because I was blaming God inside, I didn't have anything like a consistent prayer life. Even when I tried to pull myself together and say, 'You really should be praying, Holly; you really should be reading the Bible,' there was no feeling or meaning. I was just saying words.

"I was putting on a pretty good front, so most people didn't know what was going on inside the real Holly. Finally, I reached the point where I couldn't stand it anymore. I felt like I was two people. I was afraid that if I didn't seek help, I would have a breakdown or do something drastic. I prayed for the hurt to be taken away. I was honestly trying to give it up to God, but because the hurt was so deep, I couldn't do it by myself."

At last Holly made an appointment with an Episcopal priest and tried to tell him how she was feeling. When she had finished, he was silent for a while, obviously giving the matter thought and prayer. Finally, he said, "I think you need inner healing," and he offered to put Holly in touch with a trained lay counselor named Susan. Holly agreed to meet her, and they arranged an appointment in the chapel of their church.

"We set aside a little spot in the choir area and began by reading a passage of Scripture that we discussed briefly. Susan would ask me a few questions, and then we would stop and pray. First we prayed aloud, and then we listened for what God might be saying to us. During a time of being quiet, Susan said, 'Where are you, Holly? What are you remembering?' It was a childhood memory, nothing to do with the tubal pregnancy or my subsequent infertility. But it was a memory that had a lot to do with my feeling insecure and unable to measure up, to ever be good enough.

"On that occasion, I was healed of that particular childhood memory. Also, Susan was given a mental picture of me covered with Band-Aids;

the Band-Aids peeled off one by one, and the wounds underneath were healed. I'm the kind of person who needs something tangible or visual to hold onto. For Susan to receive that image in prayer, and for me to know that it was from God, was something I could cling to. From that point, I could see light at the end of the tunnel. That was the beginning."

Several weeks later, Susan and Holly met in the church sanctuary and again read Scripture, prayed, and waited before the Lord. As they talked and discussed what Holly was thinking, the hurt of Holly's tubal pregnancy came out. Susan walked her through it, asking her to go back and tell her what it was like. They also prayed over it. "In being quiet and listening before God," Holly remembers, "I began to feel that I should go over to the cross at the altar and lay this before Christ. I felt I should get up out of my seat, walk to the cross, and kneel before it or put my arms around it, and say, 'Jesus, take this hurt.'

"I sat there and thought about it, but I didn't do anything. Then Susan said, 'I think you know what you have to do. I think you have to go over to that cross and put your arms around it.' My mouth dropped open. Obviously, God was speaking through her as well as directly to me, convicting me of what I needed to do. She added, 'Only you can do it. Only you can make the decision.' I sat for a while longer, while she waited very patiently. Finally, I got up, walked over to the cross and stood there looking up at it, not saying anything, not doing anything, just looking at it.

"At last I was ready. I put my hands out and said, 'Jesus, take this hurt. I can't bear it anymore; it's hurt me too long. Take it.' I put my arms around the cross, tears came down, and it was as if a huge burden had lifted. I felt so calm and relaxed and peaceful. Peace I hadn't felt in years. The hurt was gone, and it has stayed gone. And, praise the Lord, this happened on a Sunday five years to the day it all began."

With Holly's healing came the understanding that God is principally a God of love rather than judgment. "We certainly do need to have reverence for him because he is almighty—the ruler over the entire universe," she says. "But now I see that he did not cause my tubal pregnancy or my infertility; it wasn't his fault. Yes, he allowed it to happen; he could have prevented it. But he didn't zap me and say, 'I'm punishing you for this, that, or the other thing.' We live in a fallen world, a world marred by sin, and just because we're Christians doesn't mean we're immune to bad things happening to us."

The transformation of Holly's life is evident to everyone who knows her; she radiates joy. Not only have the peace and joy that came with her healing remained, but she is now anxious to share the peace she has found with others. She says, "I know what God can do! I've experienced it. I want other people to experience this joy and not have to wait as long as I waited. I have gained compassion and much more sensitivity for other people from this whole experience, but I can't overemphasize how important it is to seek help early. My grief, unresolved for so long, could have destroyed our marriage, and it could have destroyed me."

Welcome back, Holly!

In *A Grief Observed*, C. S. Lewis says that while grief sometimes seems like a "circular trench from which there is no escape," it is really more like a "winding valley" which does come to an end.[2] When you are traversing that valley, it is as important to be as gentle with yourself as you would be with your best friend. For instance, there is no need to force yourself into situations you dread. That infant baptism, Mother's Day service, or baby shower will come off fine without you. If you allow yourself time to heal, the day will come when you can face such situations with much greater equanimity. Because of the intensity of the feelings involved, letting go and allowing yourself to grieve can be terrifying. It helps to know that grief will run a natural, fairly predictable course and that its end is not devastation but resolution and calm.

−4−

The Infertility Investigation

MOST COUPLES ARE SHOCKED WHEN THEY FIND THEMSELVES THE subjects of an infertility workup. Contraception, not conception, is on the minds of most newly married couples. Fertility is simply assumed, and the question is not "Can we have children?" but "When shall we?"

Even among the small percentage of American couples who elect not to have children, there is the assumption of choice. In fact, the effectiveness of modern birth control makes it possible for many couples to plan their families in much the same way that they project career moves or major purchases. "Five years ago," says a Massachusetts woman, "we picked out the month in which we wanted our baby to be born. I thought I was going to get pregnant the first time I tried. Never in my wildest dreams did I imagine that I might reach the age of thirty and still not have a child."

Given the almost universal assumption of being able to have children, infertility nearly always comes as a complete surprise. Kathy, a Michigan native, says, "When John and I were first married, we came up with a little package deal that was, as he says, 'neat and tidy.' He was going to finish graduate school; I was going to teach and put us through. Afterward, we would start a family. I was fascinated with his large family and thought it would be wonderful to have a houseful of children, never anticipating the responsibilities and challenges of parenthood, let alone the possibility that parenthood might not be available to us. It seemed to John and me that all he had to do was look at me with a bit of affection and, suddenly, I would be pregnant. Bingo! Well, our neat-and-tidy package deal didn't exactly work out."

Now in their forties and the parents of three sons, Kathy and John endured two traumatic miscarriages, a stillbirth, and years of waiting before the birth of two sons and the adoption of a third. One measure of the consternation their delayed parenthood caused in their extended family is the reaction of John's grandfather, the formidable patriarch of the clan who himself had fathered more than twenty children. Gravely taking John aside one day, he said, "John, what's the matter? Why, you're the first one in the family to have been married over a year and not have any children!"

Many couples methodically plan their children like John and Kathy, postponing parenthood until both husband and wife are established in careers, educational loans are paid off, and dreams of travel are fulfilled. Others are more spontaneous. Lynn, a midwesterner, writes, "For our first five years of marriage, my husband didn't want kids. His dad died when he was just six and his mom never remarried. Never having had the role model, he felt inadequate to take the responsibility of fatherhood. About three years ago, when we were considering taking over the church nursery, he looked into a classroom and saw a two-year-old boy in a bow tie, standing all alone. Something happened to my husband. He said, 'Now.' And I thought it would be just that easy." It has not been easy, however. A combination of problems makes pregnancy possible but unlikely. Now in their thirties, Lynn and her husband are facing the prospect of never having children, though they still catch themselves saying, "If we have kids someday . . ."

When surprise gives way to the need to take action and seek medical help, infertile couples quickly discover there are many conditions that can get in the way of conception and a normal pregnancy.

When Should a Couple Seek Medical Help?

Although there are Christians who believe that investigating the causes of infertility and seeking to remedy them is "tampering with God's territory," most see no incompatibility between having faith and seeking medical help. In response to the notion that medical treatment for infertility is trying to play God, one woman emphatically replies, "This is very twisted reasoning. I don't know any Christians who would tell me not to get treatment for any other medical condition. For some reason, the reproductive system is taboo. God is still sovereign, and the success of the medical treatment can certainly be left to him." She adds, "When the Bible was written, God's intervention, sought through prayer, was the only cure for infertility. Today, however, God seems pleased often to work through medical means. Statistically, an infertile couple's chance of conception increases from five percent without medical help to over fifty percent with it. Luke 11:9-10 tells us to ask, seek, and knock in order to receive; sometimes the seeking and knocking can prove long and arduous before the door is opened."

The clear consensus among those who have contributed to this book is that medical alternatives should be prayerfully and actively pursued before a couple gives up hope for a biological child. Most also agree that the pursuit of testing and treatment is a highly personal journey for which the specific direction of the Lord must be sought.

Statistics show that eighty percent of all couples who will achieve pregnancy do so in the first year of trying. (Most medical authorities define "trying" to mean having intercourse approximately every other day around the time of ovulation.) If twelve months of regular sexual relations fail to result in conception, a couple is advised to seek help. However, if they become anxious and desire to initiate an investigation within a year, there is no reason why they should not.

There are some couples for whom it is probably inadvisable to wait a full year. Couples over thirty, for example, might do well to take action earlier. In addition, women whose menstrual history is erratic, men who have had undescended testicles or adult mumps, and anyone with a history of infection or inflammation of the reproductive organs should establish the condition of their fertility early.[1]

Who Should You See?

If you cannot find a recommended infertility specialist through local referral, you can obtain the names of specialists in your geographical area by writing or calling Resolve or the American Fertility Society (see appendix for addresses). Ideally, the specialist you choose should have a practice solely or largely devoted to infertility, be associated with a teaching hospital, and have a reputation for being understanding as well as technically competent.

Why should a specialist be seen from the outset if at all possible? Infertility, a sophisticated subspecialty of gynecology, requires knowledge of endocrinology and urology and highly specialized training in reproductive physiology. Many gynecologists lack such training and are so involved with their obstetrical patients that they have little time, energy, or motivation to become informed about developments in the diagnosis and treatment of infertility. While general or family practitioners are often wonderfully supportive of their infertile patients and energetic in their efforts to help them, most simply lack the knowledge necessary to deal with cases that are other than routine.

Dealing with a doctor who is not a specialist can be costly, especially if the doctor is not honest or secure enough to acknowledge the limits of his or her competence. When Margie, a Chicago woman, became concerned about her inability to conceive, she consulted an obstetrician-gynecologist who was the darling of her circle of Christian friends. Although she was having considerable pain, her doctor told her during repeated visits that "everything felt fine." Her own reading about infertility and her awareness of her symptoms made her suspect she had a condition called endometriosis, but the doctor would take no action beyond prescribing codeine and Tylenol, drugs she felt merely masked the problem.

Eventually a friend steered her to the fertility institute associated with Northwestern University in Evanston, Illinois. After a four-month wait for an appointment, she became a patient of the director. After he examined her the first time, he saw Margie and her husband in his office and said, "I cannot tell you for sure without a laparoscopy; however, my educated guess would be that you do have endometriosis. I feel adhesions on your ovaries."

Margie says, "We knew at that point how much we had fooled around with the other doctor. The specialist was expensive but it was worth it. My suggestion for anyone with an infertility problem would be to go to someone who limits his or her practice to infertility. I wasted so much time with a doctor who was loved by many women, women who would go to no other doctor to have their babies or get checkups, but who is not an infertility specialist." Margie's advice was underscored again and again by those who have contributed to this book.

What Is Involved in an Infertility Workup?

It is not unusual to wait three months or longer for an appointment with a specialist. Once underway, the infertility workup will typically begin with establishing a detailed medical history for both husband and wife, separate interviews with each partner, and a conference in which the doctor and both marriage partners participate. Normally the doctor will then perform an internal examination of the wife and obtain an analysis of the husband's semen. In some cases, the specialist's office will handle the semen analysis; in others, the husband will be referred to a urologist.

In *Getting Pregnant in the 1980's*, Robert H. Glass and Ronald J. Ericsson report that even in so enlightened a country as France, as recently as 1979, the male factor in infertility was virtually ignored, and a semen analysis was often a last resort.[2] In this country, there is general agreement that since infertility is caused by a male problem as often as it is caused by a female problem, there is no justification for submitting a woman to a battery of sometimes painful, complicated, and expensive tests before an analysis of her husband's semen.

Once a routine internal exam has been performed on the wife and the husband's semen has been analyzed, further testing will be determined by the physician's assessment of their particular case. Although some infertility tests are conducted more routinely than others, there is no standard series.

Before proceeding too far with an infertility investigation, it is wise to determine the extent to which your health insurance will cover any diagnostic tests or exploratory surgery that may be required. I also strongly recommend that couples beginning an infertility investigation review and compare several up-to-date handbooks on reproductive physiology and infertility (see appendix). If you do so, you will be better able to follow and assess your doctor's explanations. You will also be taking an active rather than a passive role in understanding and dealing with your problem, and this may help offset the loss of control commonly felt by those who are infertile.

The following survey of the causes of infertility, diagnostic tests, and treatments is by no means exhaustive; it is offered as a primer on the complex medical aspects of infertility. The causes of miscarriage, which many believe to be the most painful form of infertility, are discussed in the next chapter.

Causes of Infertility

Female Infertility. Among the most common causes of infertility in women are:

• Infection leading to scarring and adhesions of the uterus, ovaries, or Fallopian tubes.

• Endometriosis, a sometimes painful condition in which cells from the uterine lining implant themselves outside the uterus where they "bleed" at the time of menstruation, often causing ovarian cysts, scarring, and adhesions.

• Irregular ovulation or anovulation (when ovulation fails to occur). Among the causes of anovulation is the polycystic ovarian disease known as Stein-Leventhal Syndrome.

• Cervical infection, weakness, or blockage. In some cases, polyps or unusually thick mucus make the cervix impassable.

• Uterine tumors, malformation, or extreme malpositioning of the uterus.

• Hormonal deficiencies. Insufficient progesterone production, for example, known as inadequate or short luteal phase, may permit conception but prevent proper implantation and nourishment of a fertilized egg.

Male Infertility. The most frequent causes of infertility in men are azoospermia (the absence of sperm) or sperm inadequate in number, motility (sperm swimming ability), or morphology (structure). Other causes of male infertility include:

• Sperm blockage resulting from infection or a congenital defect.

• Varicocele (varicose veins grouped in the scrotum).

• Undescended testicle.

• Adult mumps.

• Hormonal deficiencies.

• Serious injury or accident affecting the reproductive organs.

• Heat. Heat from an internal source such as a viral infection or an external source such as working around hot ovens or wearing tight jockey shorts can interfere with the maturation of sperm.

Combined Causes. In approximately one in five infertility cases, the problem is with neither the husband or the wife but with the two as a couple. Poor sperm motility combined with thick cervical mucus, for example, can result in a couple's being only marginally fertile or "subfertile." More rarely, immunologic reactions to sperm prevent conception. Sometimes there is confusion about coital timing or technique. For example, a couple may be assuming that the wife is ovulating at midcycle and timing intercourse for conception accordingly. If she has a twenty-eight-day cycle, then ovulation is likely to occur around day fourteen; but if she has a thirty-eight-day cycle, she will ovulate approximately twenty-four days after her period starts.

Some couples experience the frustration of "secondary infertility." After the conception and birth of one child, they find themselves unable to produce another. Secondary infertility may result from any of the conditions mentioned above, conditions that have developed or worsened since the couple had their child. Occasionally, complications arising from pregnancy or delivery cause subsequent infertility.

Miscellaneous Causes. Other factors that can contribute to infertility are diet, alcohol, drugs and medications, obesity, environmental pollutants, and radiation. Another suspected cause is T-mycoplasma, a bacterial organism found in the prostate gland of some males and present in the cervix or uterus in some females; the role of this microorganism in infertility is still unclear.

The offspring of mothers who took diethylstilbestrol (DES) in early pregnancy to prevent miscarriage run a higher than average risk of infertility. Most DES-exposed offspring have unimpaired fertility however. A recently discovered reversible cause of infertility is the diet and training regimen practiced by some female long-distance runners and ballet dancers; their severely reduced body fat can interfere with ovulation. Male long-distance runners may also risk reduced fertility.

The "Normal Infertile." In approximately ten percent of all infertility cases, the cause remains a mystery, and couples for whom no diagnosis is possible are often called the "normal infertile." The intense frustration experienced by those in this category is vividly captured by Tracy: "In my desperate search for fertility, I spent hours poring over magazine articles and books on infertility, searching for some magic formula or some shred of information that would enable me to become pregnant. I tried, and my patient husband endured, many so-called home remedies, such as baking-soda douches and different positions for intercourse.

"I hung out in health-food stores, reading free pamphlets and vitamin labels, spending a fortune on anything that could even remotely help me. I downed extra doses of Vitamins A, C, and E, calcium and zinc supplements, and enough herbal tea to fill a swimming pool.

"I went through three doctors, several temperature charts, countless tests, and finally, admittance to the hospital for diagnostic surgery. I had a D and C, a hysterosalpingogram, and a laparoscopy. After all of this, my gynecologist concluded that I was 'perfectly normal.' The diagnosis as written on his bill stated, 'Infertility—No Known Etiology.' Those words, imprinted forever on my mind, left me with a cold chill. 'No Known Etiology.' All those tests, all that expense, and we still didn't know anything."

Stress. In the popular imagination, stress is assumed to be a primary cause of infertility. Thus, countless childless couples have been told to "relax" or go on getaway weekends or take warm showers before retiring. One sensitive woman in her early thirties whose infertility remains undiagnosed gets regular long-distance telephone advice from her mother-in-law to "relax." The daughter-in-law says this unsought but frequently offered advice has a double implication. "First, it's my fault that I'm not getting pregnant, and second, there's something wrong with me that is other than physical."

Even some doctors, by their gratuitous advice, have helped perpetuate the myth that infertility has a psychological basis. The first doctor consulted by an Alabama pastor's wife told her, "Everything looks fine. Try to relax, get a new car, buy a house, get in debt, and you'll come up pregnant." She was later found to have such severe endometriosis that a hysterectomy was necessary.

Since there is very little scientific evidence that psychological factors influence fertility, the advice to relax is irrelevant and counterproductive. John J. Stangel, M.D., author of *Fertility and Conception: An Essential Guide for Childless Couples*, is one of a growing number of specialists who acknowledge that as medical understanding of infertility increases, psychological causes as an explanation become less and less satisfactory. They are, he says, "probably of minimal significance in the total picture of infertility."[3]

While tension is a doubtful cause of infertility, the reverse is certainly true. As Barbara Eck Menning has so succinctly stated, "The feelings of stress and frustration are the *result* of being infertile, not the *cause*."[4]

Diagnostic Tests

Test for the Male. The husband is usually asked to have a urological exam only if semen analyses show abnormalities. Since sperm count and motility can fluctuate widely, two or three sperm analyses performed over a period of time are far more reliable than one. If a urological exam becomes necessary, the physician, preferably a urologist with an interest in infertility, will check for the presence of infection, varicocele, and anatomical abnormalities. If a need for further testing is indicated, he might perform a testicular biopsy, a surgical procedure to determine if normal sperm are being manufactured in the testes; a vasography, X-ray of the vas deferentia (ducts that, if absent or blocked, can prevent the ejaculation of sperm); or hormonal and chromosomal studies.

Tests for the Female. Beyond the basic pelvic exam, perhaps the most common test for women is the keeping of a basal temperature chart. This involves making a daily record of one's temperature immediately upon waking. Ovulation is preceded by a slight rise in temperature, and keeping track of fluctuations in temperature through basal charts is a rather imprecise but often helpful means of determining if and when ovulation is occurring.

Another common test performed on women is the Huhner or postcoital test. This painless test is performed in a doctor's office within a specified number of hours after intercourse to determine if live sperm are present in the cervical mucus and whether the mucus is thin enough to allow sperm migration. If the postcoital test indicates good cervical mucus but poor sperm survival, the possibility of an immunological reaction must be considered; that is, the husband or wife may be carrying antisperm antibodies.

Other tests for females include:

• Tubal insufflation by carbon dioxide (Rubin Test), a somewhat outmoded method of determining if the Fallopian tubes are open. When women say they have had their tubes "blown," this is the test to which they are referring.

- A hysterosalpingogram is a test for tubal normalcy in which the progress of dye injected through the cervix into the uterus is monitored by X-ray. It is more reliable than the Rubin.
- Analysis of the viscosity or elasticity of cervical mucus.
- Evaluation of blood and urine to determine hormonal levels.
- Endometrial biopsy, an often painful test in which a tissue sample taken from the uterine lining is microscopically examined for hormonal evidence of ovulation.
- Laparoscopy, a minor surgical procedure involving the insertion of a lighted telescopic instrument through a small incision just below the navel, giving the doctor a clear view of all pelvic organs. Some surgeons remove small adhesions and minor endometrial implants during laparoscopy.
- Culdoscopy, a procedure more or less eclipsed by the popularity of laparoscopy, involves an incision in the vaginal wall through which a telescopic tube is inserted to view the internal organs.
- Hysteroscopy, a procedure in which the cervix is dilated and the uterus distended to determine whether there are any intrauterine abnormalities.

If a laparoscopy, culdoscopy, or hysteroscopy reveals conditions such as fibroid tumors, adhesions, or endometriosis, further surgery might be indicated. Before agreeing to major surgery, it is usually best to obtain a second medical opinion.

Treatment of Infertility

Attention to good, overall health is foundational to the treatment of infertility since factors such as poor nutrition, obesity, and alcohol abuse can all affect fertility. On one hand, successful treatment depends on whether a diagnosis is possible, the extent and precise nature of a couple's problem, and the skill and experience of the doctor or surgeon. On the other hand, the resolution of infertility is a matter for prayer, of seeking the will of God, of asking him to give the physician wisdom or guide the surgeon's hands.

Treatment for infertility is highly individual. What worked for your next-door neighbor or sister may have absolutely no bearing on your particular case. If no diagnosis is possible, a competent and sensitive physician can help a couple determine when all medical avenues for investigation and treatment have been exhausted and when it is time to say "enough."

Adoption as a Cure. Advice to adopt is almost as common as advice to relax. Well-meaning people often assert that adoption is the best cure for infertility. They invariably tell of "hopeless" cases in which pregnancy occurred only after adoption proceedings were well underway. There is only one reality behind the myth that adoption cures infertility: spontaneous cures occur in approximately five percent of infertility cases. But spontaneous cures occur no more frequently among those who adopt than among those who do not.

Treating Male Infertility. Sometimes a simple problem can be quickly diagnosed and easily remedied, saving months, even years, of anxiety. One couple we know had a son early in their marriage and waited and prayed for years, without results, for a second child. The husband is an athlete and coach who almost always wore an athletic supporter under his jockey shorts and took frequent hot showers. As a result, the temperature of his scrotum was raised to a level that significantly affected the maturation of his sperm and decreased his fertility. On a doctor's recommendation, he temporarily switched to boxer shorts, wore an athletic supporter less often, and took cooler showers. The result? He and his wife soon had a second son.

Although the answer to male infertility is occasionally as simple as switching from jockey to boxer shorts or taking antibiotics for a previously unsuspected infection, male infertility is generally difficult to treat. In cases where the reasons for azoospermia (no sperm), a low sperm count, or poor motility cannot be found, no rational treatment is possible.

However, there are promising developments in the surgical treatment of some causes of male infertility. Medical science is rapidly advancing in areas like surgical correction of varicocele or of blockages in the epididymis and vas deferentia, passages through which sperm travel. Furthermore, although only a small percentage of male infertility is medically cured, twenty-five percent of men with low sperm counts or seemingly inadequate motilities will eventually father a child, with or without treatment.[5]

Treating Female Infertility. Treatment for female infertility may be either medical or surgical, depending on the nature and extent of the problem or combination of problems. The following examples illustrate treatments available for specific conditions:

• Hormonal deficiencies, irregular ovulation, and anovulation. The synthetic drugs Clomid and Parlodel, taken orally, may be prescribed to stimulate hormonal production, which in turn stimulates ovulation. When these drugs fail, Pergonal, a costly drug that can cause dangerous side effects, is sometimes prescribed.

The media have sensationalized the multiple births associated with these "fertility drugs." Actually, there is a six percent incidence of twins with Clomid versus one percent in the general population. With Pergonal, there is a fifteen percent incidence of twins and five percent incidence of triplets.[6] Many doctors prescribe minimum dosages of these drugs to reduce the possibility of a multiple birth.

If drug therapy fails to stimulate ovulation, some doctors recommend wedge resection, an operation in which a wedge of tissue is removed from each ovary. Although there is a high rate of ovulation after this surgery, the reason for its success is unclear.

• Endometriosis. Endometriosis may be treated medically through the prescription of birth control pills or danazol (Danocrine), both of which suppress rather than cure this disease. Extensive endometrial implants call for surgical removal.

• Cervical factors. There are douches to neutralize overly acid cervical secretions; antibiotics are available for cervical infections; and thick cervical mucus may be helped by added estrogen. Artificial insemination with the husband's sperm may be employed if sperm are unable to bypass a cervical barrier.

• Blocked Fallopian tubes. Like endometriosis and anovulation, blockage of the Fallopian tubes may be treated either surgically or nonsurgically. According to Glass and Ericsson, a hysterosalpingogram has a therapeutic effect on the tubes when administered with an oil-base rather than water-base dye; they claim that fertility is enhanced for six or seven months after this procedure.[7] Another nonsurgical means of attempting to open the tubes is hydrotubation or tubal lavage, a controversial procedure in which the tubes are flushed with a sterile solution.

Rapid advances in laser and microsurgery—delicate surgery using a microscope and very fine suture—also offer hope to women with blocked tubes. Although this surgery sometimes is spoiled by scarring that occurs after the operation, it can—if successful—remove tubal adhesions. Also, it is now technically possible to remove a damaged section from a tube and rejoin the healthy ends. Success depends largely on the extent and location of the blockage.

Artificial Insemination, *In Vitro* Fertilization, Ovum Transfer, and Surrogate Motherhood

Artificial insemination, *in vitro* fertilization, ovum transfer, and surrogate motherhood are four controversial alternatives that, despite broad and often sensational media coverage, are presently available only on a limited basis to childless couples. Some Christians find none of these options acceptable; others see the new medical technology as an answer to their prayers. Following is a brief survey of these four practices and some of the key issues involved in each of them.

Artificial Insemination. There are two kinds of artificial insemination: artificial insemination using the husband's sperm (AIH) and artificial insemination using the sperm of an anonymous, unrelated donor (AID). Most donors are medical students or residents who are paid a modest amount for their services. Although some artificial inseminations take place privately, the majority are performed by physicians. Artificial insemination rarely "takes" on the first attempt, but if conception is going to occur, it usually happens within six or seven cycles.

AIH, where the husband is the donor, is indicated in only a few circumstances; the most common case is a cervical or vaginal barrier to the deposit or migration of sperm. Although many Christians dislike the clinical nature of AIH and would of course prefer conception to occur through intercourse, none of those with whom I have talked would rule it out if it were their best or only hope for conception.

AID, where the donor is not the husband, is a different story. Although a number of those who have contributed to this book find it acceptable and several have tried it, others equate it with adultery. (In the official teaching of the Roman Catholic Church, it *is* adultery.) They grant that it is a passionless, clinical form of adultery, but insist that it is adultery nonetheless.

Not all Christians agree. Recently, a Christian couple in my community, reluctant to risk transmitting a known genetic disorder through the husband's sperm, opted for AID after a careful review of the ethical issues involved. The husband, who happens to be a seminary student, did not keep their decision confidential, and many of the Christians with whom he shared it were openly incredulous and disapproving.

Typical of those who feel moral and physical revulsion toward AID is a Pennsylvania woman who says, "Because my husband's sperm count is zero, artificial insemination would have to have been by donor. To let you know how repulsive that was to me, I considered it nearly equal with being raped. I couldn't put aside the fact that I would be carrying a child by a man other than my husband. Someone trying to persuade me in favor of AID said, 'Once you bear the child, the fact that it was conceived by another man's sperm will be erased.' Someone else said she would rather carry a child she knew was at least half theirs than raise a child that, biologically, wasn't theirs at all. I can't agree."

As this woman's comments suggest, two of the advantages claimed for AID are a biological relation to the mother and the opportunity for her to experience pregnancy. The flip side of that is that impregnation of his wife by another man's sperm and the loss of his own genetic continuity can be extremely difficult or impossible for the husband to accept. The advantages of AID are further offset in the minds of some by: (1) unsettled questions about the legal status and rights of AID-conceived children (only fourteen states have laws protecting the rights of children so conceived); (2) the possibility of transmitting disease or genetic disorders through donor sperm, despite screening; (3) the remote possibility of inbreeding resulting from a marriage between two unwitting AID offspring fathered by the same donor's sperm.

Other issues include whether to tell an AID-conceived child about his or her beginnings, what psychological effect that information might have, and whether it is right to cut a child off from half of his or her genetic heritage. Owing largely to the decrease in the number of children available for adoption, AID is gaining in popular acceptance. In the United States, approximately 10,000 children are conceived by AID annually. Because of the volatile issues inherent in AID, many clinics and physicians offering this service require couples to undergo counseling before being approved for artificial insemination.

In Vitro *Fertilization. In vitro* means "in glass," hence, the coinage of the term, "test-tube baby." The four major steps in *in vitro* fertilization include: (1) retrieval of the egg(s) through means of laparoscopy; (2) precise timing of the retrieval during the menstrual cycle; (3) fertilization of the egg(s) in a sterile dish; and (4) placement of the fertilized egg(s) into the uterus. The last step is the most difficult to accomplish successfully. This very delicate procedure results in a live birth approximately fifteen to twenty percent of the time.[8] *In vitro* fertilization is generally used in cases in which the husband's sperm count and motility are normal and the wife has blocked Fallopian tubes.

Because a child conceived through *in vitro* fertilization is the product of the husband and wife and involves no third party, many find it less controversial than AID. To those who believe that life begins with conception and is sacred from that moment, the most troubling aspect of *in vitro* fertilization is the fate of those eggs that are fertilized but not implanted. Sometimes more than one egg is implanted in the hope that at least one will survive; sometimes "extra" fertilized eggs are discarded; sometimes, partly to avoid the ethical issue, they are frozen for possible future use. An additional concern with *in vitro* fertilization is the fear that manipulation of the egg and sperm outside the body may result in birth defects. So far, this does not seem to be the case. In 1979, the Ethics Advisory Board of the Department of Health, Education and Welfare found no ethical problems with *in vitro* fertilization.[9] Whether or not there are ethical issues to consider in *in vitro* fertilization, there are some sticky legal questions. For instance, in 1989, the disposition of frozen fertilized eggs became a hotly contested issue in a widely publicized divorce settlement.

Ovum Transfer. For nearly a century ovum or embryo transfer has been used in animal breeding, but only recently has it been successfully accomplished in humans. In July 1983, doctors at the Harbor-UCLA Medical Center announced the first successful ovum transfers in human history. From among a group of fourteen donors, five fertilized ova were retrieved and two pregnancies achieved. The procedure requires precise timing and involves artificial insemination of a volunteer fertile woman with sperm from the husband of an infertile woman, retrieval of the egg five days later, and placement of the egg in the uterus of the infertile woman. Because the husband's sperm is used, a child so conceived obviously has a biological relationship to him. Another advantage claimed for ovum transfer is that it enables an otherwise barren woman to experience pregnancy, hence prenatal bonding with the baby, and delivery. Because of the involvement of a third party, some opponents of ovum transfer see it as an adulterous practice. Many who would not define ovum transfer as adultery still question the morality of experimenting with fertilized human ova, and in the United States, government funding for such research is prohibited.

Surrogate Motherhood. In principle, surrogate motherhood is simple: out of altruism or for material gain a woman agrees to bear a child for an infertile couple and is artificially inseminated with the husband's sperm. In practice, it is fraught with a host of ethical and legal questions.

What if, as in the widely publicized case of Baby Doe, a child is born handicapped and all parties disclaim it? What if the surrogate mother finds it impossible to relinquish the child, something that has already happened in several cases? Among other potential complications, there is the possibility that the surrogate mother who decides to keep the baby and sues the putative father for child support could win the court battle. What of the potential for exploiting surrogate motherhood for financial gain? Fees as high as $25,000 have been proposed. Many opposed to surrogate motherhood see it as a practice that reduces human life to a commodity that is bought and sold.

Some argue that surrogate motherhood and the refinement and practice of *in vitro* fertilization, AID, and ovum transfer should be left entirely to medical and legal authorities. I disagree. Some, including several of those who have contributed to this book, say, "What could be wrong with any means that would provide a desperate couple with a child?" Again, I disagree. Because infertility is such an emotional issue and there is such pain for childless couples, concern for what is right can become lost in what is expedient. An unfulfilled desire for a baby no more automatically justifies acquiring one by any available means than an unfulfilled sexual desire automatically justifies four bare legs in a bed.

A recent television program about genetics featured a couple who have a child conceived through AID. During their segment on the show, the wife said, "I didn't think of it as someone else's sperm; I just thought of it as a way that we could get a baby." Similarly, doctors who promote AID are quick to present it as "ethically indistinguishable from a blood donation."[10] As Christians who believe that life is not merely a product of chance but created by God and therefore sacred, we cannot afford to duck the hard questions inherent in controversial alternatives for the childless. They demand honest, clearheaded, and prayerful consideration.

Such consideration does not necessarily mean rejection of all these alternatives by all Christians who weigh them, but it should at least help us proceed carefully and remember that before God, each individual life has significance even before birth. As David wrote in Psalm 139:

> You created my inmost being;
> you knit me together in my mother's womb.
> I praise you because I am fearfully and wonderfully made;
> your works are wonderful,

I know that full well.
My frame was not hidden from you
   when I was made in the secret place.
When I was woven together in the depths of the earth,
   your eyes saw my unformed body.
All the days ordained for me
   were written in your book
   before one of them came to be.

Some are quick to dismiss talk of the sanctity of individual human life as mere religious mumbo-jumbo, but as C. S. Lewis has written in his essay "Man or Rabbit?" the Christian takes a radically different view: "To the Materialist things like nations, classes, civilizations must be more important than individuals, because the individuals live only seventy odd years each and the group may last for centuries. But to the Christian, individuals are more important, for they live eternally; and races, civilizations and the like, are in comparison the creatures of a day."[11]

When to Say "Enough"

Despite the discomfort, awkwardness, and sheer bother of the infertility investigation, testing and treatment offer not only hope but solutions to many. Although they have firsthand experience of the pain, inconvenience, and expense of an infertility workup, the overwhelming majority of those who have contributed to this book recommend seeing the infertility investigation through. Today, successful diagnosis and treatment are possible in more than half of all infertility cases. And a carefully chosen doctor, who is understanding as well as technically competent, can do much to ease the emotional and psychological strain.

Although many infertility cases are happily resolved, knowledge of the causes of infertility is incomplete, and often an investigation can drag on without resolution for a very long time. In such cases, a couple must eventually decide when to continue the testing with its stress, expense, and diminishing possibilities for a return and when to say "enough."

Personal limits must also be set as to which medical alternatives are acceptable and which are not.

One Christian couple, professionals in their early thirties, found themselves among the ten percent for whom the cause of infertility remains a mystery. After many months of prayer and waiting, the wife wrote to her gynecologist, who is an eminent infertility specialist, "I put so much energy and worry into wanting to get pregnant that my life is passing me by. We have not spent any time planning for our future because we keep hoping it will include a child, yet we have no way of knowing whether it will. Therefore, we have come to a decision. I no longer want to think about temperature charts, progesterone levels, the timing of sexual relations, or Clomid. I never want to go through the tension involved in all of this only to be devastated when I get my period.

"No doubt there will always be a part of me that still hopes—a sequestered longing to be a mother. I'm sure there will be times when I will wonder if my husband regrets not being a father. And sooner or later I'll have to deal with thoughts of growing old without children or grandchildren.

"But we've made a decision to change our focus, and we think that's best for us at this point. We will at least make a concerted effort to stop dwelling on why."

–5–

The Pain of Miscarriage

S TRICTLY SPEAKING, MISCARRIAGE IS NOT A FORM OF INFERTILITY; those who miscarry are obviously capable of conception. Yet they share the same fate as those who are childless through infertility, and they know similar emotional and psychological distress.

For a few unfortunate couples, miscarriage becomes almost commonplace with repetition. A midwesterner who has had six consecutive miscarriages and has never carried a pregnancy to term says, "Pregnancy has become like a disease that I have for a short time and then get over." For others, losing a pregnancy is an event that helps them decide that childbearing is not for them.

For most who miscarry, however, a failed pregnancy is a painful loss—a death to be mourned. It sharpens rather than decreases the desire for children. One woman recalls, "Up until that first miscarriage, I could have honestly said I could be happy with or without children. After the miscarriages, and partly because of my emotional investment in them, it became intensely important for me to have a child."

In words with which many who have miscarried can identify, Edith Schaeffer recounts the loss of her own "much wanted baby": "I had the sadness of a miscarriage at three and a half months. Far from a hospital, in a chalet in the Alps, I had to lie for some hours with that tiny baby beside me—with its threadlike fingers and toes, the ears beginning to form, the arms and legs, curved body, and curled-over head—still connected with me, as the doctor waited for his instruments to come up on the late-afternoon train. I wept for the cut-off life, and I had an incredible desire to push it back into me, to give it a chance to grow. . . . A senseless idea, an impossible desire. It was a death to me."[1]

The idea that miscarriage, especially early miscarriage, is loss of life rather than mere loss of tissue may seem fanciful or sentimental to some. Over 1,500,000 abortions are performed in the United States annually. Yet to those who lose a desired pregnancy, a miscarriage is not the end of an anonymous embryo; it is the death of a child for whom plans have been made and to whom individual characteristics, such as a name, have been applied—from the first days and weeks of life.

In words typical of many who have miscarried, a Pennsylvania woman says, "Even though that red tissue didn't look like much, holding it in my hand was like holding a child. I remember all sorts of questions going through my mind: Did this child have a soul already? What did the good Lord want us to do with the remains? Can the doctor just take it and coldly put it under a microscope?"

Questions like these are common, and long after couples have borne other children, many remember those lost through miscarriage with quiet regret. They remember the pregnancies they have lost as real people, as actual lives, not just tissue. Although it is true that most women who miscarry will go on to have one or more normal pregnancies, this in no way cancels out the pain.

Miscarriage: The Physical Event

The unintended termination of a pregnancy before the twentieth week of gestation—"miscarriage." This is the layperson's term for what the medical profession calls "spontaneous abortion" (in contrast to "induced" or "therapeutic" abortion). Naturally, many couples are stunned by the use of the emotionally charged word "abortion" to describe the end of a greatly desired pregnancy.

Miscarriage is surprisingly common. In their excellent book *When Pregnancy Fails,* Susan Borg and Judith Lasker note that each year some 800,000 American families are affected by miscarriage; like most experts, they estimate that fifteen to twenty percent of all recognized pregnancies end in miscarriage.[2]

A miscarriage typically begins with vaginal spotting, which may be brown at first and turn to bright red if bleeding continues. Since vaginal bleeding occurs in some normal pregnancies, it is not always a sign that miscarriage is inevitable, but bleeding during pregnancy should always be taken seriously. Continued and increased bleeding, accompanied by cramps, is an ominous sign of imminent miscarriage. The cramps of miscarriage are actually labor contractions that cause the cervix to open and expel the embryo, and the unexpected strength of these contractions, combined with possibly heavy blood and tissue loss, can be frightening.

There are several types of miscarriage. In a "threatened abortion," a woman bleeds and may have cramps, but her cervix remains closed. The miscarriage becomes an "inevitable abortion" if, in addition to continued bleeding, the cervix dilates and contractions begin. In a "complete abortion" no tissue remains, and the cervix closes; in such cases dilation and curettage (D and C) are not ordinarily required. (The D and C is usually performed in a hospital under general anesthesia. It involves opening the cervix and inserting a loop-shaped instrument into the uterus to scrape away unexpelled pregnancy tissue gently.) "Complete abortions" are rare after the eighth week.

"Incomplete abortion" occurs when the fetus and placenta are not entirely expelled; when tissue remains, a D and C is essential to prevent hemorrhaging. In a "missed abortion," the fetus dies four weeks or more before being expelled. Upon the embryo's death, symptoms of pregnancy subside and a pregnancy test would prove negative. "Habitual abortion" is the rather chilling term used to describe three or more consecutive miscarriages.[3]

Another type of miscarriage occurs as a result of ectopic or tubal pregnancies. Tubal pregnancies represent an estimated one percent of all pregnancies. Future medical developments may make it possible to transplant an ectopic pregnancy to the uterus, but at present an ectopic pregnancy always ends in miscarriage. Signaled by vaginal bleeding and lower abdominal pain beginning about two weeks after a missed period, a tubal pregnancy is very difficult to diagnose and often goes unrecognized until it has ruptured the Fallopian tube in which it is implanted, causing a serious medical emergency. Because surgical removal of the tube in which the fertilized egg has lodged is the usual outcome of an ectopic pregnancy, it not only results in miscarriage but also in decreased fertility.

Unless a miscarriage happens quite early, it will take time for a woman's body to catch up with the event. A swollen abdomen and enlarged breasts, once evidence of the life within, are now hollow reminders of a pregnancy that is past. Once the fetus dies, hormone production will drop off sharply, possibly contributing to biochemically based mood swings. As Rochelle Friedman and Bonnie Gradstein point out in *Surviving Pregnancy Loss*, this hormonal reduction is a physiological stress that hits precisely when a woman is not only physically but emotionally vulnerable.[4]

Causes of Miscarriage

Many couples mistakenly blame themselves for a miscarriage and painstakingly review their lives in search of a cause. Husbands often ask, "Why couldn't we have refrained from sexual intercourse during pregnancy?" And many wives blame themselves for working too hard or exercising too vigorously.

Yet none of these normal activities is believed to cause miscarriage. The fetus is suspended in a virtually shockproof environment, and it would take a severe jolt to harm it. Nor are anxiety and nervousness believed to cause miscarriage, except in rare cases of psychological trauma such as might result from a serious automobile accident. Miscarriage is almost always biologically rather than psychologically triggered. Furthermore, rarely can anything be done to thwart a miscarriage once it has begun.

To the intense frustration of many couples who want to understand the "why" of a miscarriage, it is not always possible to determine the cause. As with infertility in general, there is still much about miscarriage that is not understood. There are several known and suspected causes, however, and these are briefly summarized below.

Genetic. Approximately one-half of all spontaneously aborted fetuses are abnormal. Because many first-trimester miscarriages are due to genetic errors, there are many who conclude miscarriage is "nature's way of getting rid of her mistakes," a cliché that is small consolation. Most genetic defects result from random abnormalities in a particular egg or sperm or in the irregular distribution of chromosomes when the fertilized egg divides.[5] Such abnormalities are unlikely to be repeated. Only in rare cases are chromosomal abnormalities inherited from the parents; and usually only after three first-trimester miscarriages is a couple encouraged to seek genetic counseling.

Inadequate or Short Luteal Phase. After ovulation, a structure called the corpus luteum produces progesterone, which, in turn, acts on the endometrium or uterine lining, preparing it to receive and nourish a fertilized egg. In luteal-phase defect, an inadequate level of progesterone prevents proper implantation and growth of the fertilized ovum. In the past, this condition was often treated with progesterone supplements. The effectiveness of this treatment has been called into question, and it is now believed that added progesterone during early pregnancy might harm the fetus.

Uterine Malformation, Fibroids, or Adhesions. A uterus divided into two cavities by an extra wall (separate or bicornate uterus) does not always lead to problem pregnancies, but if the division is severe and the fetus lacks adequate room to develop, miscarriage will occur. Distortions of the uterus caused by fibroid tumors or by Asherman's Syndrome (a condition in which overly vigorous curettage, or scraping, of the uterus has caused adhesions) have also been implicated in miscarriage. Surgery can sometimes correct these problems.

Immunologic Factors. It is a great biological mystery why the fetus, which has inherited one-half of its genetic material from its father and is to that extent a "foreign body," is not rejected by the mother's immunologic cells. An assumption presently under study is that protective antibodies normally produced by a pregnant woman make it possible for the mother to carry the fetus; when breakdowns in this protection occur, miscarriage results.

"Incompetent" Cervix. When a cervix is weak through congenital defect or, as is more common, through a tear resulting from previous pregnancy or surgery, cervical dilation occurs too early under the weight of the fetus and miscarriage quickly follows. A cause of many "late" or second-trimester miscarriages, cervical weakness can often be corrected by tightening the cervix with sutures made after the first trimester and left in place until labor begins.

Drugs and Environmental Causes. According to Glass and Ericsson, one-half pack of cigarettes per day or one ounce of alcohol twice a week have been associated with an increased incidence of spontaneous abortion.[6] Caffeine is another suspected cause. Other factors contributing to miscarriage are radiation, particularly if the fetus is exposed before the twentieth week of gestation, and chemical pollution of the environment.

As an example of the effects of chemical pollutants, Borg and Lasker cite the unusually high rate of miscarriage, stillbirth, and birth defects around the Love Canal area near Niagara Falls, New York, where toxic wastes had been dumped for years, contaminating the water supply. They also cite the high rate of miscarriage experienced by Oregon women in the late 1970s when the areas where they lived were sprayed with 2,4,5-T, a herbicide containing dioxin.[7] DES (diethylstilbestrol) exposure has also been associated with a higher than average risk of miscarriage, tubal pregnancy, and stillbirth.

Infection and Disease. The microorganism T-mycoplasma, which may be treated with antibiotics, has been found in couples with histories of recurrent miscarriage, but its precise role in miscarriage is unclear. German measles (rubella) is a known cause of both miscarriage and birth defects. Diabetes and lupus erythematosis, a disease that affects the body's connective tissue, are also believed to be causes. *Maternal Age.* For unknown reasons, women under twenty and over forty run greater than average risk of miscarrying.

Miscarriage: The Emotional Impact

One woman who has experienced two miscarriages and a stillbirth says, "Miscarriage is the most painful form of infertility in its roller-coaster effects; you're exhilarated with the knowledge a baby is growing and devastated when its existence is terminated." Part of the trauma of miscarriage is the feeling that your body is going wrong. Those who miscarry often wrestle with doubts about their physical adequacy and femininity.

Her first miscarriage left Kathy greatly shaken. She asked herself, " 'What is wrong with me physically?' I remember looking at myself in the mirror—staring at my pelvis and hips—and saying, 'Now, look, you are meant to have children. You are strong and healthy. You have always been strong and healthy. Now, really, there is no reason in the world why you should have difficulty carrying children.' "

Partly because miscarriage happens in their bodies, most women who miscarry believe that they have been more affected by it than their husbands. While most husbands do not feel the same attachment to the baby that the wife experiences, many do feel considerable disappointment and sadness. Miscarriage strikes the couple, not just one partner, and because attention is often focused on their wives, husbands may feel overlooked and puzzled that few seem to realize the miscarriage is their loss, too.

Usually a husband's first concern is the health and well-being of his wife. Believing that he must be strong for her, he may keep the lid on his own feelings, and his reaction to the miscarriage may consequently be postponed until weeks or even months later when he suddenly feels strangely irritable, anxious, or sad. Unfortunately, when a husband tries to be strong for his wife's sake, his apparent stoicism can be misinterpreted as a lack of feeling or caring. Many wives wistfully say they would be comforted and feel less alone in their grief if their husbands could more freely express their own sorrow.

Since the grief of miscarriage is dimly understood by the larger society, a couple may find that others—hospital staff, friends, family—fail to recognize the significance of their loss and offer little help by saying the miscarriage was "for the best" or that they "can always have another baby." Others may simply leave them alone in their grief. "When my mother hinted that I should have children," one woman sadly recollects, "I told her I had miscarried three times. She turned her head away, saying, 'That's not something to talk about.' She didn't mention the subject again for months."

In the face of such reactions, a couple may wonder if their response to their loss is irrational and begin to question their emotional and psychological stability. Nevertheless, grieving is a legitimate response to losing a desired pregnancy. Even though a couple may have another child, it is normal for them to feel the loss of the one who might have been. The need to grieve, find comfort, and take time to heal after a miscarriage is borne out in the following accounts.

Sue and Ken

"When the doctor used the word 'infertile' to describe my condition," Sue recalls, "that was a real shocker. I remember walking back to the car and crying there for a while before I could drive home." Irregular ovulation combined with a short luteal phase severely reduced her chances of conception. Sobered but also challenged by their physician's diagnosis, Sue, a nutritionist, and her husband Ken, a chemist, approached their problem as scientists. For five years they carefully kept charts of Sue's basal temperature and ovulation. "Our record keeping," Sue acknowledges, "may have been one way of coping, of trying to manage the problem."

They eventually located an infertility specialist, an endocrinologist whose logical, scientific approach they liked. After reviewing their copious basal charts, he agreed that there were problems with ovulation and the luteal phase. His next step was to prescribe the minimum dosage of Clomid. Sue describes herself as "the sort who is reluctant to take aspirin for a migraine," and she responded cautiously. Before filling the prescription, she researched Clomid's possible side effects by asking her brother-in-law to Xerox the relevant pages from his medical school textbooks for her. She soon became convinced that Clomid was a reasonable intervention, and after only three months on that drug, she conceived.

"I was very excited—thrilled—but even before the pregnancy test, I was spotting. My doctor ordered me to stay off my feet, and because I was teaching that was difficult. I was torn. I wanted to do what I could to preserve the pregnancy, but I also had a sense of obligation to my job. My mother used to push me out the door with a box of Kleenex and say, 'Go to school. If you don't have a temperature, you're not sick.' My tendency is to believe that life won't go on without me if I'm not there."

Finally one Friday night, after Sue had submitted herself to fourteen weeks of unaccustomed inactivity in an effort to save the pregnancy, severe cramps signaled its imminent termination. "Even up to the end I hadn't made the full connection that the pregnancy was over. In the hospital, they wanted to give me Demerol, and I said, 'If it will in any way hurt the baby, then I don't want it.' I was still clutching at hope.

"One reason this miscarriage was so trying is that I really thought of this child as a person, something I had a hard time communicating to my doctor. I remember asking, when I had the D and C, if there was anything particularly aberrant about the fetus. That showed a misunderstanding on my part as to what a D and C is, but it also showed him how much I expected the baby to have identifiable characteristics.

"After the D and C, I was lying in a room stuck off down at the end of the maternity floor, thinking about what happened. I visualized chunks of tissue, which was the child I had nurtured for fourteen weeks, chunks of tissue, which were to be disposed of. Almost concurrently, I saw that child with Christ; and the knowledge that someday I will see that child is very comforting." In committing her unborn child to the Lord, Sue, like many Christians who miscarry, found solace in Psalm 139, in which David writes, "All the days ordained for me were written in your book before one of them came to be" (Psalm 139:16).

While recovering, Sue was fortunate to have the support of her husband and discerning friends. Ken told her, "If we never have children, that's okay. You're important to me, and you're enough for me." For Sue, that relieved the pressure. Also, while she was in the hospital, she was visited by two friends who had miscarried. "They didn't say very much," she recalls. "When I was somewhat glib and said that after the uncertainty of the previous fourteen weeks I was relieved the pregnancy was over, they knew my initial response would change to grief. They quietly said, 'We're here if you want to call and talk.' During the following weeks, they telephoned Sue frequently and sent notes, and she gratefully remembers their being simply and quietly present. Rather than offering her the usual clichés, they listened.

Sue says there are some things her friends were wise enough *not* to say:

"Well, God knows what is best."

"Better that things end now than to find out later that there's something wrong with the baby."

"You can always get pregnant again."

"You know, I have a cousin who couldn't get pregnant for years, then she miscarried three times, but now she has four kids."

Sue adds, "These kinds of statements are well-intentioned, but not at all consoling." Others who have miscarried agree. As one woman says firmly but without rancor, "It did not help me at all to have somebody with two perfectly healthy children and who had given birth with no problems say, 'I know what you must be feeling.' I didn't think she did. And even though I thought to myself, 'At least I can get pregnant,' it didn't help me to hear that from somebody else."

In addition to having a supportive husband and friends, Sue also discovered several other resources, including writing poetry and keeping a journal. "As soon as I suspected I might be pregnant, I began keeping a journal of my thoughts and poetry. I treasure those poems today. After my miscarriage, I continued writing. 'Journaling' was useful in organizing my thoughts and identifying feelings that I needed to express. Also, at times when it was difficult to pray, writing down my thoughts and reflections often took the form of prayer."

Another step Sue took toward coping with her miscarriage was resolving the question: "If I don't have children, then what am I going to do with my life?" "Out of my miscarriage," she says, "came the realization that my life could not be on hold while I waited for a child. I knew I had to deal with the possibility that I might never have a child. I didn't want to continue teaching, and I certainly didn't want to just sit around and mope." In her typically thorough and systematic fashion, Sue wrote down job ideas under the broad heading of "home economics," her major in college. She came up with seventeen possibilities to investigate. After narrowing down her interests to nutrition, she investigated graduate courses and explored volunteer opportunities. "That gave me a focus," she says. "There is a real tendency to live in tomorrow and miss today. I didn't want to do that."

Still another resource that Ken and Sue discovered was participating in a weekly Bible study with just two other couples. Each couple was asked to express one significant, personal need that the group could focus on as a prayer concern. Finding themselves in an atmosphere of mutual support, Ken and Sue were free to voice their particular concern and were encouraged by the knowledge that others were praying. "It was also comforting to recall God's faithfulness in past situations," says Sue. "In studying passages of Scripture like Psalm 77, I realized that although the path of God's people is not always clear and sometimes leads through the sea—through turmoil and uncertainty—the Lord is there, leading his flock."

Today, Sue's infertility is happily resolved, and she and Ken are the parents of two small sons, Timothy and Andrew. Now thirty-three, she has traded the frustration of infertility for the considerable demands of two preschoolers and is in the unaccustomed position of having to be concerned about birth control. While her infertile years are behind her, she says, "Although I wouldn't want to go back to those years, I wouldn't want to cancel what I learned from them either."

Out of Sue's pain came increased compassion for others. When she worked as a hospital dietitian, she was alert to patients admitted for "threatened abortion." She prayed for them, kept informed about their condition, and if she felt it was appropriate, she sent a note of encouragement. Today she has a ministry of prayerful concern among friends and neighbors for whom children have not come easily. "During the discomfort of my last pregnancy, a pregnancy complicated by circulatory problems, I tried to remember that there were people who would endure almost anything for the hope of carrying a pregnancy to term. I asked the Lord to give me a clearer vision of those people so that I would have a better perspective on my own distress."

Sarah and Bert

"For the first eight years of our marriage," Sarah recalls, "we happily postponed having children. There were things we wanted to do. Finally, we had been on two study trips to Europe, Bert was established, and I had that rare commodity—a part-time teaching job that would enable me to combine work and children. Plus, I was nearing thirty." Sarah expected that it would take time to conceive, but she thought, "If not this month, then next." After about six months, however, she dreaded getting her period.

After more than a year of trying to conceive, Sarah had what seemed like a normal period, except that the bleeding didn't stop. She continued spotting for weeks. Since the same thing had happened once when she was in college, she didn't think that much about it. Finally she called for a doctor's appointment, and she was surprised when the nurse said she would have to have a pregnancy test before the doctor would see her. It had never occurred to her that she could be pregnant and still have a period. She was absolutely flabbergasted when the pregnancy test proved positive and she discovered she was about eleven weeks along.

"When I saw my doctor he was very cautious. He said that women who spotted could go on to have fine pregnancies but that I should be aware that the pregnancy could end in miscarriage. He told me to rest and explained what to expect if I actually began miscarrying—that the brown spotting would become red and I would start having cramps. In that sense, I was prepared. In actuality, my mind refused to accept the possibility that I might miscarry. Within twenty-four hours I had names picked out and my maternity wardrobe planned. I knew what I was going to do for childcare, and I had mentally rearranged the house to provide for a nursery. The baby was a reality. Within a week, I had miscarried.

"Although we had told few people I was pregnant and the miscarriage came as a shock to everyone at church, I experienced an outpouring of support. The rector's wife and the assistant rector's wife came over right away and told me that they both had miscarried twice. Not only had they experienced the same kind of loss, but since they had children at that point, they also represented hope. While they didn't actually say, 'You will grieve,' they told me to expect a recovery period. One said, 'It was several months before I stopped crying.' Because I work in a high school where I hear all the time about girls who have abortions or put their babies up for adoption, the miscarriage just didn't seem fair. I think that if I had not had the support of Christian friends, it might have been easier to get angry at God."

The difficulty of Sarah's first miscarriage was compounded by a trying hospital stay. "I had a D and C, and when the doctor had done some scraping, he abruptly showed me a basin of material and asked, 'Is this what the other stuff looked like?' Later, two staff members wheeled me to my room in the maternity ward. One of them was obviously pregnant, and all the way up in the elevator, she patted my stomach and said admiringly, 'Isn't that nice and flat?' She obviously didn't know what had happened to me, but that was very difficult."

Like Sarah, many women find that hospitalization for miscarriage is one of the most disconcerting aspects of the whole experience. Husbands, too, often find it difficult, especially when they are separated from their wives, a circumstance that can leave them feeling useless. Because miscarriage can happen without warning, a couple may not have time to think and exercise some control over the hospital stay. Friedman and Gradstein suggest that when it is possible to make specific requests rather than merely acquiesce to the hospital staff, there are several steps that can make a hospitalization less painful: (1) Insure that husband and wife have reasonably free access to each other; (2) request a private room, preferably located somewhere other than maternity; (3) discuss with the doctor in advance of the D and C whether to see the fetal tissue and how it will be disposed of.[8]

Because a maternity floor is considered "clean" and women are believed less likely to pick up another patient's infection there, it remains the ward where most patients who miscarry will be located. However, a well-trained hospital staff will make every effort to screen a woman having a miscarriage from those giving birth and will locate her where she and her husband will come into minimal contact with new parents and their babies.

When Sarah miscarried a second time, she found that the attitude of the physician and other medical personnel can make an enormous difference. "When I went to my doctor's office for a checkup," Sarah recalls, "he was just wonderful. He said, 'I've just come from a conference on miscarriage, and do you know, we don't even understand what makes a woman keep this foreign body—a pregnancy—nor do we understand what causes labor to start to expel it.' That helped me. I realized that any birth that goes to full term is a miracle and that I couldn't be too surprised if some don't make it.

"When my doctor added that he hadn't run any test on the embryo because he didn't consider miscarrying a problem until after the third, I started to cry. He came over and put his arms around me and said, 'Don't cry. If you cry, I'll cry.' I could tell he understood what a loss it was for me, and he also reassured me that not only had I done nothing to cause the miscarriage, there was nothing I could have done to prevent it."

Some months after her second miscarriage, Sarah became pregnant for a third time. For the first time, she felt truly pregnant. Like many women who miscarry, she did not have the usual symptoms—fatigue, morning sickness, and breast enlargement—in her first two pregnancies. This time, Sarah went on to give birth to a precocious daughter named Sasha who shares her dark hair and eyes. "Sometimes I think that if that second pregnancy had gone to term, I never would have had Sasha. When I think of how perfect she is for us—she is exactly the child we wanted— then I can think maybe, just maybe, that's a clue to why the miscarriage happened."

Sarah and Bert's daughter Sasha has peopled her lively four-year-old imagination with a hundred sisters and thirteen brothers, many of whom she has named. She would very much like a real brother or sister. With a smile, Sarah says, "I try to make it clear that babies come small, that you can't play with them right away." With respect to trying to have another child and giving Sasha the brother or sister she is lobbying for, Sarah says, "I believe I have to be prepared for the possibility of miscarriage, and I haven't been willing to subject myself to the emotional strain while Sasha was small and needed so much attention. Only within the last six months or so have I felt ready to be pregnant again."

Several weeks after our interview, Sarah told me that the day on which we had talked was the very day she had begun to suspect she might be pregnant. Upon reaching age thirty-seven, she delivered Joshua, a healthy baby boy. Although Sarah's struggle to bear children is over, she, like Sue, remains sensitive to others for whom children have not come easily. Both remind those who have lost a pregnancy that recovery takes time.

Sue says, "For fifteen to eighteen months after my miscarriage, Friday nights were more difficult than other times of the week. I wasn't consumed with grief during that time, but I was conscious of anniversaries. This year was the first that I didn't remember October twenty-seventh, the date on which my miscarriage occurred." Sarah adds, "About eight months after the first miscarriage, Bert and I were sitting in a restaurant, and a man walked in with his little girl. There was something about the sight of those two people together that got to me; I just started crying. Also, during a whole year after that miscarriage, baptisms were very difficult; I can remember a couple of times when I had to leave the service. Don't feel bad about grieving," she concludes. "Don't feel bad if it seems to take a long time."

Miscarriage: Bearing One Another's Burdens

Stepping Stones editor Leslie Snodgrass says, "Having lost a baby through miscarriage myself, I remember the need for comfort. Although I don't profess to have all the answers (and although needs differ from person to person), I offer these suggestions:

"Don't avoid a loved one who is hurting simply because you are afraid you won't know what to say! The Lord gives us grace and wisdom for each moment, and the feeling of being alone and forgotten during such a difficult time only adds insult to injury.

"Don't assume your friend doesn't want to talk about it! Chances are, she does. I have found that talking about it, reliving the details, helps one face the reality of the loss. This is an integral part of the healing process. You can't assume she does want to talk either; you must be sensitive to what she says (or doesn't say).

"If she does want to talk about it, let her! Often, those with the best intentions find themselves filling in an awkward moment by recounting their own personal tragedies, blurting out suggestions, or throwing out scriptural reminders without allowing the person in need to get a word in edgewise. Listening is key. In listening, you will be able to discover what your friend's special need is. What is she having trouble coping with? The loss itself, why God allowed it to happen, whether it is wrong to be angry?

"Don't assume you have all the answers to her questions (or feel inadequate if you don't!). You may not have the answer because the Lord wants your friend to find it in him. Miscarriage often leads to feeling alone, abandoned, or angry. The insatiable need to know the 'why' to a myriad of questions will draw her into the arms of the only Person with the answers that relieve the pain.

"Do remind her she is loved and thought of often. You don't have to camp on her doorstep to show her you care. She may be physically worn out and need time alone. Pray for insight into creative ways to show her you care. For example, a ready-to-heat meal is a blessing after a hospital stay, and a flower stuck in the mailbox with a note attached is a pleasant surprise.

"Don't use clichés. Clichés like 'Time will take care of it' may or may not be true, but more often than not they sound callous and insensitive.

"Do continue to be sensitive to your friend's loss in the months that follow. In my own case, it took a while for the initial shock to wear off. When it did, I was left with an incredible emptiness. I needed to be constantly reminded that the Lord loved me, and that he hadn't forgotten me. My loss was made more difficult because it had taken me a long time to get pregnant. It took several years to get pregnant again, and special friends and family continued to pray. I was sustained by those prayers." (Adapted with permission from "Miscarriage: Bearing One Another's Burdens," *Stepping Stones,* October 1982.)

–6–

Living without Children

"Childfree" or "Childless"?

WHEN THE INFERTILITY INVESTIGATION LEADS TO A DEAD END, OR when pregnancy repeatedly ends in miscarriage, couples must eventually ask themselves: Do we adopt or remain childless? For some that is a knotty question. For others there really is no question; initiating adoption proceedings seems a natural, almost inevitable step.

What of those who do remain childless, who neither adopt nor ever have biological children? Do they become isolated, embittered people, or can they embrace life and affirm the love and faithfulness of God?

Childlessness is not a hopeless condition. Yes, there is loss in being without children. But there are also possibilities. Just as being a parent is an art and an adventure in which the outcome cannot be foreseen or predicted, life without children can also be a journey in faith.

And childlessness is a legitimate option to consider whether or not a couple eventually pursues adoption. As one person who now has an adopted son says, "Once it is apparent that you cannot have biological children, it is important to reconsider whether you really do want children. Give yourself time. Make sure you're not just following convention.''

Making the Decision

The most obvious factor influencing the choice to adopt or remain childless is the decline in the number of babies available for adoption. Although some adoptions are completed within two years, five-year waiting lists are not uncommon; the potentially long wait combined with the high cost of some adoptions can be daunting. The frequent job transfers and relocations common in our mobile society can also affect adoption plans. One couple, affiliated with a well-known international evangelistic organization, moved eight times in eight years, making it impossible for them to see adoption proceedings through. Some couples who are unsure about adoption simply postpone the decision indefinitely; years pass by and one day they realize they have decided more or less by default.

Elements such as intuition can also affect the choice to adopt. The decision to have a baby is more than a solely rational choice, more than a calculated adding up of the pros and cons of parenthood, and the decision to remain childless is not reached by logic alone. For example, a midwestern couple in their thirties says, "We believe in, encourage, and support adoption but have never been more than mildly interested in it for ourselves. The expense and the fact that we live in an apartment that does not permit children have been excuses for not investigating any further, but with sufficient motivation we would have tackled these obstacles." While they have an intuitive sense that adoption is not for them, this couple would be hard-pressed to give objective reasons why. "Our only explanation for this," they say, "is that God doesn't seem to have led us in that direction yet." Each couple interprets the will of God and decides what is best for them through different and sometimes complex combinations of influences and circumstances. Among the subtle forces that can affect our thinking about children are: social pressure to conform to the traditional family model; our perspective on marriage and family; a fear of growing old and dying alone; and our particular sense of vocation.

Pressure to Conform

The common assumption that to be childless is to be selfish and immature puts considerable pressure on infertile couples. Since others often assume that childlessness is by choice, a couple may think they need a child to prove they are responsible adults rather than perpetual adolescents. Yet the logic that parenting is selfless by definition and childlessness intrinsically selfish has always escaped me. Many of the reasons people give for having children are obviously self-interested rather than altruistic.

Furthermore, while the family is certainly an ideal place for learning and practicing love and self-sacrifice, it is not always such a haven. The family can also be an insular, greedy institution, unaware of the needs of those beyond the biological circle and bent everlastingly on feathering its own nest. Similarly, some who are childless undoubtedly use their freedom for self-indulgence, while others forego extravagance in order to invest themselves and their resources freely in the lives of others.

There is an obvious correlation between the circles in which we move and the amount of social pressure placed on us to become parents. For example, a woman who is putting her husband through theological seminary says, "The majority of the couples I know in the seminary community have become pregnant within the past two years. In this environment, getting pregnant is seen as the thing God expects us to do next. The tacit assumption is, 'What else could there be?' "

"During my year on the seminary wives association board, I was the only one of the eleven board members who didn't either have a baby or get pregnant. Even our adviser, who is well into her thirties and has a thirteen-year-old son, got pregnant by a fluke! During the last board meeting of the year, we met to socialize, and the entire evening's conversation was about babies. I realized that, in the absence of a set agenda, that was all we—or they—had in common. Although I miss the fellowship of those women, I was relieved when my term on the board was over."

Some find enormous pressure within their churches to conform to the traditional family model. At one church meeting the preliminary topic of conversation was the number of babies being born in the parish. A man looked directly at one childless couple and stopped the discussion by saying loudly, "Well, what's the matter with you guys? When are you going to get with it?"

Seldom is the pressure so direct; it more often takes the form of unintentional exclusion. As one woman says, "Our church has been having its own baby boom, and every time I turn around somebody else is pregnant. Before a service or during the coffee hour, I often find myself standing in a group where someone starts talking about their kids or about yet another person who is having a baby. Because I'm experiencing something completely different, it's as though a wall has been thrown up. Eventually, I turn and slip away because it hurts too much."

My husband and I discovered that pressure to conform depends to a considerable extent on where you live. When we left graduate school, we went to a Pennsylvania college town where the population numbers fewer than 8,000, where the nearest bookstore is twenty-five miles away, where the only newspaper is a thin, twice-weekly edition long on advertisement and short on news, and where the most heralded event in recent memory was the coming of a McDonald's restaurant. Roles for men and women tend to follow fairly traditional lines in that community. At parties, for instance, women cluster in the kitchen talking breast-feeding and recipes, and men remain in the living room discussing college affairs and sports.

All of this was rather new to my husband and me, since we were raised in the suburbs of major cities. But even though we knew small-town life would require some adjustments, we were looking forward to it. We bought our first house, a solid old place with a postage-stamp-size yard, and began to settle in.

Before we were completely unpacked, a faculty wife, who had warmly welcomed us to the community, came for morning coffee. She had hardly arrived before she blurted out, "I can't tell you how out-of-it I felt here before Jamie was born." She knew nothing of our circumstances, and she could not have guessed at the impact of her words. I think she was simply trying to identify with me. Yet as I listened to her describe the family orientation of the town and her sense of being outside the mainstream until she became a mother, my optimism about our move was suddenly clouded. It had been less than a year since I had discovered my infertility, and I was still trying to find my way. I thought, "Don't tell me that the one thing I *must* do to have a place in this community is the very thing I *can't* do."

On the whole, my husband enjoyed his work in the mathematics department of the college, and my position in the college public information office allowed me enough latitude to continue work on a book then in progress. We both enjoyed the fellowship of a couples' Bible study, and I made a wonderful, understanding Christian friend who had experienced years of infertility. The two years we spent in western Pennsylvania were by no means a dead loss. They were busy and productive.

But the apprehension raised by my first acquaintance was not altogether unfounded. As the months passed and we returned from occasional trips, we found that the closer we got to home, the more subdued we both became. We felt hemmed in by the provincialism of the place and shut out from most of the town's life that was largely centered in the schools and church youth programs. We also felt somewhat circumscribed in our jobs since possibilities for increased responsibility were quite limited. Since we did not want to gad from one place to another in a vain search for the ideal situation, we decided to sit tight, pray, and wait for direction.

During our second year in that small town, my husband was invited to apply for a position at Gordon College, a Christian liberal arts college near Boston. That opportunity seemed tailor-made for us, and when Dick was offered the job, we did not hesitate to accept it. Only when we began making plans to move to Massachusetts did we fully realize how entrapped we had begun to feel. In retrospect, I believe the Lord showed us a clear path out of an environment that had become stifling for us. Incidentally, two weeks before we received word of the opening at Gordon, we were spending the Christmas holidays with my parents. During a seemingly inconsequential after-dinner conversation, my mother asked us where, out of all the places we had traveled, we thought we would most like to live. Our answer? The Boston area.

We are now in our tenth year on Boston's North Shore. No, it is not the Promised Land. Real estate would be less expensive in the Promised Land.

But it's close. I can still hardly believe our good fortune in living here. We again live in a small town and a comfortable old house with a handker-chief-size yard. But here the population is far more heterogeneous than in western Pennsylvania. Naturally, the PTA, church youth programs, and Little League are all integral parts of community life. However, nearby Boston and the surrounding towns offer many cultural events, greater professional opportunities for both of us, and wider possibilities for ministry. In short, there are many more people whose circumstances are similar to ours and there is much more room to breathe and grow.

What is the point to this story? Is it that childless couples should flee small town and rural or semi-rural environments and head for more cosmopolitan places? Not necessarily. While that Pennsylvania town was a way station on our particular journey, a childless couple with a less urban background than ours and different vocational interests might have easily called it home.

The point is that our surroundings can have a major impact on how we as individuals cope with our childlessness. The norms and attitudes prevailing in our particular church, neighborhood, and town are extremely influential. In the case of fertile women, one study has shown a direct correlation between a woman's rate of childbearing and that of her three closest friends.[1] Those of us who are infertile are no less susceptible to social influences, and it is wise to explore whether our restlessness and longing arise from the absence of children or from other circumstances. A wish to conform socially is not a good reason to adopt; it is important to evaluate how much this wish may be motivating our desire for children.

Marriage

Another form of social pressure placed on childless couples is the sugges-tion that something is missing from their marriage until they have repro-duced or at least adopted a child. If a couple believes their marriage is incomplete without children, they will naturally find it difficult to envision a future without them. Yet in spite of the close relationship between the institutions of marriage and the family, the marriage relationship has a separate integrity of its own. And children are not necessary to justify that union or the love expressed within it.

Despite our sexually open and "liberated" society, I suspect that some unconsciously think that procreation sanctifies sex, which they believe is somewhat tainted, even within marriage. As Catholic thinkers Mary Perkins Ryan and John Julian Ryan point out, "The idea that sexuality is an unfortunate aspect of human nature, redeemable only by repression and non-use, has strongly influenced Christian teaching from Patristic times to our own. The original impetus for such a negative attitude seems to have come from outside Christianity, from the Stoics and others disgusted with the licentiousness of their times. Christian teaching has, indeed, always argued for the basic goodness and redeemability of matter, of the body, of marriage and procreation. Nevertheless, distrust of sexuality has predominated through the centuries."[2]

One of the church fathers responsible for this distrust of sexuality is Augustine; he thought that original sin was transmitted from one generation to the next through lustful aspects of intercourse. Believing that childbearing was the sole end of marriage and sex, Augustine taught that the use of contraceptives was wicked. Sex, intrinsically bad, could be cleaned up only by parenthood. Later teachers such as Martin Luther affirmed sex within marriage as a good gift of God and found no biblical basis for Augustine's unfortunate but once widely held view.

For most Christians today sex serves more than strictly biological ends. "The biological purpose of an organ or a system is not its only purpose. Eating and drinking, for example, can serve many psychic needs as well as physical ones; eating and drinking together can foster a whole range of human values other than strictly biological ones."[3] Apart from solely procreational purposes, sex can obviously bond two people together and serve as a powerful vehicle for the expression of love. There are many good reasons to adopt a child, but legitimizing a marriage and sex is not one of them. Marriage, not children, sanctifies sex.

The reality that procreation is not the sole end of marriage is difficult for some to grasp. "My husband is sterile," one woman wrote, "and since my reason for getting married was to become pregnant and raise a family, it is very difficult for me not to scream at him, 'It is all your fault we can't have children. I'm leaving!' " She added, "I feel stuck in a relationship that can produce no life." I replied that only on the most literal level was their relationship incapable of producing life. For I am convinced that a reasonably whole and healthy marriage can be a gift of grace to others, whether or not children come. A sound marriage can provide an emotional home into which others may be welcomed and nurtured.

In addition to having students in our home on occasion, my husband and I have taken several summer study trips abroad with undergraduates. During those trips, we live in close quarters with some thirty students for eight weeks at a stretch, and it would be impossible to miss their intense interest in our relationship. How courteously do we address each other? Is there real warmth between us? Do we work in harmony or at cross-purposes? Many of these students come from fractured family situations, and they are keenly interested in what makes our relationship tick. By God's grace we offer them a healthy, though imperfect model, and our marriage becomes a gift to them.

These students return from time to time. They appear at our door to introduce their spouses, show off their babies, or tell us about their first homes. Some want advice on graduate schools or jobs. In a sense these students and graduates have become our loose-knit, extended family, a family in which there is certainly life.

My husband and I are hardly exceptions. There are many childless couples who enjoy richly rewarding marriages. Often those who do go on to adopt express regret over not making more of their childless years. They wish they had placed more value on their time alone and made better use of it.

In words that many infertile couples will find affirming, the late Christian counselor Walter Trobisch addressed childless marriages. Speaking to an African audience, he quoted Genesis 2:24, "Therefore, a man leaves his father and his mother and cleaves to his wife and they become one flesh." Trobisch then asked how this verse ends, and a man replied, "With a full stop," or period. Trobisch emphasized this "full stop," noting that in that key verse about marriage, a verse quoted four times in the Bible, there is not a word about children.

"The effect of these words on my audience was tremendous," he recalled. "It was as if I had thrown a bomb into the church." For in the culture of those to whom he was speaking barrenness is sufficient grounds for divorce. "Don't misunderstand me," he continued. "Children are a blessing of God. The Bible emphasizes this over and over again . . . Children are a blessing to marriage, but they are an additional blessing to marriage. When God created Adam and Eve, he blessed them and then he said to them: 'Be fruitful and multiply.' From the Hebrew text it is clear that this commandment was an additional action to the action of blessing. Therefore, when the Bible describes the indispensable elements of marriage, it is significant that children are not expressly mentioned. Leaving, cleaving, and becoming one flesh are sufficient. Full stop . . . The full stop means that the child does not make marriage a marriage. A childless marriage is also a marriage in the full sense of the word."[4]

Family

Another factor which can have a bearing on whether we can confidently and optimistically envision a childless future is our view of family. Some argue that a couple can be a family. For example, one woman says, "It hurts when people refer to children as 'family.' Two can be a family too!"

To others, a family without children is a contradiction in terms: "To me a family is more than two people. In my view, we were not a family until we adopted Jeremy. We were a lonely couple. Even during those times when we felt, 'Sure, we can make it as two,' I still had a real loneliness in my heart. A family meant sharing our lives with children."

Still another says, "I share so much more with my friends than with my relatives that I see my friends as my 'real' family." This woman, like many who are separated from their biological connections by geographical, emotional, or spiritual distance, finds that her primary relationships, her 'family' relationships, are with friends rather than relatives.

Some who are childless find great comfort and security in their ultimate identity as members of the larger family of God. Within the body of Christ, they find many brothers and sisters, mothers and fathers, and children and grandchildren. Although they would have welcomed children, they discover they do not need children—whether biological or adopted—to have a sense of family connectedness or belonging. No useful purpose would be served here by trying to establish whether a particular view of family is "right" or "best." Rather, the point is simply that our perception and experience of family will help determine how vital it is to have children of "our own."

Growing Old and Dying Alone

A very real though seldom spoken concern of those contemplating a childless future is the fear of growing old and dying alone. As one woman tearfully told me, "I'm afraid—and perhaps this is selfishness on my part—I'm afraid of growing old and not having children. What would I do if I don't have children to take care of me like I intend to take care of my mother?"

Many living in nursing and retirement homes can testify that having children is not a guarantee against a companionless old age. Many lonely elderly people have children who do not visit them or include them in their lives in any way. Nevertheless, for most of us the thought of having our children and grandchildren near us as we grow older and perhaps more dependent is as comforting as the prospect of being alone is disconcerting. Several of those who have contributed to this book have come to terms with this fear.

For example, Nancy, a Pennsylvanian now in her fifties, says, "I used to be concerned about being lonely in my old age when my friends and relatives were enjoying their children and grandchildren. I've come to grips with that and have decided that the Lord has provided for me very well up to this point. Why wouldn't he provide for me in my later years? I'm not ready to retire yet, but I'm looking forward to having some free time for pursuits that the demands of my job have forced me to put aside. Perhaps God has given me interests such as gardening and handwork to supplement my life so that I'll never feel lonely."

Marjory Bankson, whose story is told in the next section, "Choosing Childlessness," also speaks to the fear of growing old alone. "I'm forty-three, and my husband is forty-four. Since he is a typical Type-A personality, I fully expect to outlive him. Several years ago, in a time of imagining what it would be like to have no children and to be alone as an old woman, I caught a glimpse of myself old and poor in a county home somewhere, dying in a hospital bed. That was not where I wanted to be but where I was. In the middle of that vision or picture, I saw a practical nurse by my side as I gradually sank into a coma and then into death.

"Then an extraordinary thing happened. I realized that my picture of my own dying had much more to do with my reaching spiritual completion than with whether children were at the bedside. The other piece of that image was the presence of that nurse, an older woman I didn't know. What that figure told me was that if I do my work now, freely giving and receiving love, somebody will be there when I die if that's what I need. I can trust God to be God, and to provide from the abundance of his universe and not my biological family."

Vocation

In writing of a turning point in her experience, a West Coast woman says, "Once, in the early morning hours, I prayed to the Lord for understanding. Suddenly, I knew he was present. He asked me to see myself giving my children to him, and I had a vision of his taking those children from my arms. When I released them, I saw how much he loved and cared for them. Then he said, 'If I choose to give these little ones back to you, then you will know it is my will. If I do not, I promise to fill the void in your life.' That was the answer to my anxiety."

Our sense of calling or vocation can play a central role in filling the void of which this woman speaks. For some women, no other vocation can begin to substitute for motherhood; they simply cannot imagine life without children. Others who were once terribly disappointed by their infertility have discovered great fulfillment in varied and sometimes unlikely callings. A children's ministries director in California says, "Life is so ironic. Do you know what I'm doing? I'm leading parenting classes! I can offer my education and my heart for families, and the women have lovingly accepted me, not caring that I don't have children. God does work in unexpected ways!"

Nancy is among the many who have found that the assurance of God's love and a full life do not depend on having children. For the past thirty years, she has invested in the lives of others. For twenty-three years, she was the Christian education director of a large Pennsylvania church where she was loved by both the young people and their parents. At a time when she questioned why she didn't have any children, the kids at church would say, "Oh, you don't need any. You have all of us!" For the past seven years, Nancy has been a director of student affairs at a liberal-arts college. In that capacity she has counseled, befriended, and mothered hundreds of undergraduates.

Nancy was by no means untouched by her infertility. At a particularly low point after the death of a family pet, she cried, "Everybody else is having babies, and I can't even have a dog!" Yet her clear sense of calling kept her from despair. She says, "I knew that I was going to go into some kind of Christian service when I was in the eighth grade. Since I have always felt that God had something in mind for me that was different, I wasn't consumed with grief the way I might have been if I had another kind of vocation. Having a routine nine-to-five job would have been one thing, but because of the nature of my work, I realized our childlessness was part of God's plan. In fact, I was so busy with my work that I really had no time to dwell on the subject of our infertility. I was too full of happiness serving the Lord!

"When I entertain the notion that I have missed something in life, I think about all the blessings I have enjoyed that others have missed. I am most blessed!"

Nancy has a well-defined vocational interest. What of women whose occupations have simply been fill-ins between marriage and motherhood? Can they, too, imagine life without children?

Although the answer is clearly "yes," finding a new source of direction usually takes time. Fae, a missionary returned from India, would be quite content to be a full-time mother, but being childless has forced her to reevaluate her calling. She was awaiting her second surgery when she wrote to me, "I am again facing the question, 'What will I do with my time—with the rest of my life—if I don't have children?' Tears come when I face the possibility of a future without a child, but I've been strengthened through reading good books and seeking the Lord. I have realized my husband and I are a family and that there are many good and fulfilling things to do even without children. My days have been filled with visiting people, evangelism, gardening, studying the Word. . . . There is so much to do for God without children."

There is indeed a rich variety of possibilities before those of us who remain childless. Depending on such factors as our particular gifts and financial circumstances, we might elect to live on one income so that one partner might devote his or her time to work that is worthy but poorly compensated. Another model is suggested by a professional couple I know who, for many years, have been the mainstays of a church where there are many financially strapped students and few well-paid professionals. In addition to giving generously of their income, this couple also has a ministry of hospitality to scores of foreign students. Still another model is suggested by an older couple who have taken early retirement to prepare for lay ministry. The wife, a secretary, and the husband, a carpenter, have both worked throughout their adult lives. Nearing sixty and having achieved a modest measure of financial security, they wish to give their later years to serving the local church.

At whatever stage we happen to be in our lives, a question to consider in making vocational choices and changes is: How can we as individuals and as a couple best express our God-given gifts and fulfill the call that is uniquely ours in Christ? While our desire for children might have been frustrated, our hope for full and productive lives certainly need not be.

Choosing Childlessness

Many Christians see having children as a given, as something that is expected of them as Christians. A few, however, elect not to have children because of commitment to a demanding vocation or for other legitimate reasons. In making this choice they risk criticism, even ostracism, from their fellow Christians.

In *Freedom of Simplicity,* Richard Foster notes that while having children is clearly the norm, voluntary childlessness is a legitimate option and calling for some Christians. He is one of the few Christian leaders with the courage to say this aloud. "To be sure," Foster says, "some have made the decision (to forego having children) from purely selfish motives; but others have done so in order to be free to care for the children of the world. I am very close to a couple who have consciously chosen not to have children so that they may have a more effective ministry among teenagers. Their home is open to young and old day and night. Although one night in their home is enough to drive me crazy, I must confess that their ministry is an extraordinarily effective one."

Foster adds, "A couple must be in covenant unity with one another in any decision of this nature. This is no place for a husband to try to exercise some kind of 'headship' over the wife. Such a decision takes time. The feelings of each spouse must be given full expression. At no time should there be conveyed a sense of spiritual inferiority if children are desired. This is a matter of calling, not spirituality."[5]

One couple who have taken the less-traveled route of which Foster speaks is Peter and Marjory Bankson. Although their circumstances are different from most who have contributed to this book, their response to the call of God is valuable for those of us who are infertile and contemplating the future.

Marjory is a potter and teacher who ministers to many through both Faith at Work and the Church of the Saviour in Washington, D.C. She and her husband, Peter, a retired career military officer, elected not to have children because Peter's position required long absences on sometimes dangerous duty, absences that would have left Marjory a single parent for considerable stretches. For most of one five-year period, for example, Peter was either in the war zone in Viet Nam or in the hospital recuperating from his two tours of duty there.

In reflecting on their decision not to have children, Marjory says, "I look first at the life of Jesus and second at the life of Paul the apostle. Then I look around me at women who have chosen a religious vocation, many of whom never marry, many of whom choose celibacy. And I see that the higher call—the call to love and the call to servant ministry—is the longer range and larger calling for each of us. I also look around at friends who have children, and I see the amount of time and energy and sacrifice that being a parent requires, especially since we don't determine the form, the intellect, even the biological immunities that children bring into the world. I watch friends whose children are not healthy or not fully functional in our technological society, and I see that their ministry must of necessity be to one or two persons."

Marjory adds, "I really see the reason why the apostle Paul urged men and women to remain unmarried in favor of their religious calling. The time and energy required for a family are enormous, at least for the kind of parenting I would want to do. When a ministry began to open up for me—a ministry I never cultivated but which simply grew—I saw that if I had children I couldn't have gone off to do church workshops and leave children home with a baby-sitter. Not having children began to be very freeing for me. I can go to women who have children; they cannot come to me.

"Also, our house has become a feeding place for what my mother-in-law used to call our 'stray people.' Many of these people are young, single, professional women working in the Washington area who know that because we don't have small children, they really are free to come if they need a place to cry. I think of myself as a safe place, a refuge, for young women who are trying to find their way. This is a place where my mothering is coming out, and my sense of calling to this ministry goes back to seeing myself as part of God's larger family, a family of faith.

"It seems to me that the model Jesus gave us begins with exploring who we are, exploring our gifts and skills, and exploring being in relationship with others. There is a poignant scene when Jesus is teaching and his mother comes to the door. She knocks and asks him to come back home, in a sense asking him to be more ordinary by the familial standards of her culture. He refuses to go to the door, and he says, 'Who are my brothers and sisters but the people who do the will of God?' It seems to me that he is saying there are conventional expectations placed on us by our culture and primarily by our mothers, and one of the first tasks of his followers is to separate from those ordinary expectations and really examine their unique call.

"As I let go of those routine expectations of repeating the patterns of my mother and grandmothers, I open myself to the unique calling that is mine. I think this often gets clouded for women who feel an inner urge for *something*. Instead of staying with the unknown of what that is, they fill up that urge with a pregnancy. I have seen this many times as women approach forty, and I think that to hold off or to explore what being childless means may indeed be a deeper spiritual path."

As Marjory's words suggest, "vocation" and "calling" convey much more than merely "job" or "career." These terms encompass our whole orientation toward life. For most of us, our vocation includes being parents. For some of us, it does not, and we must find other avenues for nurturing others and expressing our creativity. In either case, before we rush to fill up an inner void with a child, we need to take time to listen and hear the word of God for us.

–7–

Adoption
Chosen Children

"T HE PROSPECT OF ADOPTION COMFORTS ME," WRITES A WISCONSIN woman. "I do not have to bear a child to be a mother. If there is a reason for the pain of infertility, perhaps it is that God has a child out there who needs us."

Similarly, a Massachusetts woman says, "I couldn't understand why God picked me, someone who loves children so much, not to bear them. I felt I was being punished for something, but I didn't know what. One night a friend asked, 'Did you ever stop to think that the reason may be that God knows that you could take an adopted child and love him?' That hit me! I had never thought of it that way, and that was the thing that was most comforting to me."

Like many whose desires for a biological child seem destined to go unfulfilled, these women have found hope and a possible explanation for their infertility in adoption. Even though adoption has become more difficult in recent years, it does indeed remain a bright alternative for those seeking a child to love and call their own.

Among the many couples for whom adoption has been an answer to prayer is Paul, a printer employed by a hospital, and his wife, Linda, a rehabilitation nurse. "In many ways, Matthew, our special gift from God, has been a healer of pain," Paul says. "He is a special little boy who has brought new life to his grandparents as well as to us."

At the church dedication of their son, Paul recalled their experience of infertility. "As four years went by, we became increasingly frustrated, bitter, and depressed with our infertility problems. We asked, 'Aren't we good enough? Don't we give enough? Don't we try enough?' We asked ourselves these questions, and we asked many other Christians and no answers came. We over-ate and over-spent to try to fill the void in our lives. . . . In making resolutions for 1981, we decided that one of the things we were going to try to do was understand our spiritual selves better." Linda adds, "About this time we accepted our infertility, and I decided I was going to have no other gods before me. We moved on to focus on letting God have his will in our lives. The Word started to make sense; I saw relationships healed; and I began to see signs of happiness and joy return to our lives."

After four years of pursuing medical treatment for their combined infertility problems, Paul and Linda began to consider adoption. First, they spoke with a pastor who had assisted in several adoptions, and he advised them to tell everyone they knew that they were interested in adoption. Then, at a Resolve symposium, they saw "Trying Times: A Crisis in Infertility," a film in which the main character sends letters about her interest in adoption to many friends and acquaintances. Next, Linda read *Beating the Adoption Game* in which author Cynthia Martin advocates telling everyone you know that you are looking for a baby.

Linda was intrigued by this nontraditional approach to adoption, but Paul was skeptical. Although private adoption is legal in their state, Paul's first reaction was, "If we were to do it ourselves, it wouldn't be kosher." He gradually warmed to the idea, however, and concluded, "God would not have given us this strong desire for children had he not wanted us to have any. Despite being discouraged by several well-meaning friends, we acted on faith. We decided to send out a letter and see what kind of miracle God might stir up."

On Mother's Day weekend, they signed and addressed more than 250 printed copies of their final draft and sent it to fellow church members, Paul's colleagues, and Linda's nursing friends. The following is the abbreviated text of that letter:

It seems appropriate that the freshness and excitement of spring should bring this letter to you, for it is with much excitement that we are sharing our desire for a family.

While we will continue our infertility treatment with the goal of having a child "naturally," we want you to know that we are open to adoption. Recent trends in birth control and abortion have drastically reduced the number of infants available for adoption, and many experts now feel that one should go about adopting in some rather "creative" ways.

The way we have chosen for now is to let our friends and family know that we are prayerfully considering this possibility. It is so exciting to consider that God might work in such a miraculous way as to use a family member, a friend, or church or business contact to let us know of a child who may need a family.

We are asking that you do two things:

—Remember our desire for a family faithfully in prayer.

—Keep us and this letter in mind and pass it on to someone else you know who might be able to help us.

We feel that adoption—not abortion—is God's way, and since we have been adopted into his family (Romans 8:14-17), adopting a child into ours would follow quite appropriately.

Please join us in prayerful watching.

Printed beneath the text of their letter was a paraphrased promise from Psalm 113 that they claimed for themselves: "He gives children to the childless." The response to their letter was an immediate outpouring of support from friends and acquaintances, and only six weeks after it was mailed they received the phone call that led them to their adopted baby. In October of 1981, they became the parents of Matthew Aaron, a four-day-old infant. Even more remarkable is their adoption in October 1983 of Michael Andrew, a second infant referred to them as a result of their Mother's Day letter.

Today, Linda and Paul see their bright-eyed little boys as "visible answers to prayer." They remain active in Resolve out of a desire to help others deal with infertility, and they are quick to encourage the pursuit of private adoption. The subject of several newspaper and magazine stories, they say, "Because God has been so good to us, we feel strongly obligated to share our experience."

Adoption Alternatives

As anyone who has looked into adoption is aware, Paul's and Linda's experience is hardly typical. Few adoptions are arranged so quickly. In the case of traditional agency adoptions, for example, simply getting your name on a waiting list often requires perseverance. If you succeed in finding one or more agencies whose lists are "open," you may wait many months, even years, before being invited to take the first step of filling out an application.

Once your name reaches the top of an agency's list, your patience will be tried still further. After being assigned to a caseworker, you will be asked to participate in a home study. The home study varies somewhat from agency to agency, but it normally involves a series of interviews designed to get acquainted with you, assess your suitability as adoptive parents, and prepare you for the adjustments of the adoption itself. The term "home study" is somewhat misleading, since only one interview actually takes place in your home; the others are conducted at the agency. After the home study is complete and you have been approved, you must wait until the agency locates a child who appears to be a good match for you.

The prospect of a long wait is understandably disheartening to couples who yearn for a child, but those who stick it out find their patience amply rewarded. As Teri Yates, an Oklahoma mother of an adopted daughter, says, "We discovered that adoption can be a discouraging, frustrating process, but the end result is worth all the anxious waiting. Our first angel is now three years old, beautiful, easy-going, and highly intelligent. We confess we're proud and doting parents. Since she could have had any parents, we feel privileged. The Lord chose her just for us!" Teri is active in the Tulsa chapter of the Oklahoma Council on Adoptable Children. "When I counsel prospective adoptive parents, I tell them not to give up in frustration but to keep plugging and try every possible avenue."

The adoption picture varies considerably from one geographical area to another. While attempts to adopt through an agency may lead to a dead end in your city or town, private adoption may be possible in your case just as it was in Paul's and Linda's. Private, or independent, adoption is legal in all but six states (Connecticut, Delaware, Minnesota, Michigan, Massachusetts, and North Dakota). It typically involves a doctor or lawyer who acts as an intermediary between a childless couple and the birth mother. Many take the first step toward private adoption by contacting ministers, obstetricians, and lawyers to introduce themselves and express their interest in locating an adoptable child.

Private adoption is a perfectly legitimate alternative, but those pursuing it should be careful to have sound legal counsel and to deal only with intermediaries whose integrity is established. In independent adoption, the only legally permissible expenses are a reasonable fee for professional services and the health-care and delivery expenses of the birth mother. A request for fees that seem excessive may well be an indication that you are flirting with the illegal and highly risky black market in adoption.

Jane, a New Yorker who has a son adopted through legal private channels, says getting involved with the adoption underground is much easier than one would expect. "During the emotional aftermath of infertility," she says, "many people will do anything for a child. A friend of mine made a contact in Georgia. When she called, the contact said, 'Sure, we can help you. You can have a baby in three weeks. Just come down with $6,000.' She and her husband were so excited, they didn't even stop to think. Friends cautioned them and, upon investigation, it turned out they had been in touch with a black market ring. The emotional state you're in makes you vulnerable to such traps."

Owing largely to the scarcity of adoptable American babies of any race, many who wish to adopt infants are turning to international adoption. Over the past decade, according to Resolve's adoption fact sheet, more than half of all children adopted in Massachusetts have come from countries like Colombia, Haiti, India, and Korea. A number of agencies specialize in such adoptions, which require agency approval and a home study as outlined above. International adoption is frequently complicated by bureaucratic red tape and inexplicable delays in the country of origin. Nevertheless, it is a promising alternative for many.

Although international adoption often represents a couple's best hope of adopting an infant or very young child, it is not for everyone. As one couple says, "We knew we could get a Caucasian infant if we were willing to wait, and we decided we could deal best with a child whose background was as close as possible to our own. We talked about adopting a baby from a Third World country, but we decided that a child from another country has a culture he needs to know. We didn't think we were capable of giving a child that other culture. It was a question of being honest with ourselves."

Others are able to accept the implications of ethnic and racial differences. Dennis and Nancy adopted a Colombian infant through the Alliance for Children. "We knew that a white American baby was probably unrealistic since we were already in our thirties, and we wanted to get on with it. The thought of adopting from another country never bothered us. Because Colombians do not adopt their own, many orphaned or abandoned children live in deplorable conditions there. To us, it is simply wonderful that our longing for a child is being fulfilled and that we can provide for a baby who desperately needs a home. Among the issues our home study forced us to address was how we were going to respond to a dark-skinned child. We were not at all repulsed by the prospect; we just wondered how we would feel about it when the baby was actually in our arms." The home study helped Dennis and Nancy think through and resolve such questions.

Like Dennis and Nancy, many who adopt internationally are just as excited about it as they would be about a pregnancy. Jeannette has an adopted Korean daughter and a biological daughter who, to her amazement, was conceived when she was nearly forty. She couldn't understand all the fuss over her pregnancy. Friends were enthusiastic about her 'becoming a mother,' but as Jeannette says, "I was already a mother!" Similarly, Tracy says, "Once I started dealing with infertility constructively, my husband and I began to look into adoption. We found a Christian agency that places Korean children, and we are now awaiting the arrival of a Korean baby girl. To me, waiting to meet that airplane from Korea will seem like being in labor. I recently finished decorating the nursery, and my eyes grow misty every time I enter that room. Only now the tears are happy ones. I know that this baby will be as much a part of our family as a 'natural' child would have been."

In addition to international adoption, there is the possibility of adopting "special" or "hard-to-place" children. Such children are usually either in a sibling group that must be adopted together, older than six, or disabled in some way. Since "special children" often need experienced parents and frequently do best in homes where there are other children, it is the rare childless couple who represent a suitable match for them. Nevertheless, it is an alternative worth exploring. A particularly good resource for those considering adopting older or other special-needs children is *No More Here and There,* Ann Carney's warm, down-to-earth account of adopting an older child (see appendix).

Foster care is another option. Although many dislike the impermanence of foster care, some see it as both a ministry and a means of testing their interest in parenting. Foster care often amounts to short-term crisis intervention, but there is a trend toward "permanent foster care," which involves the guardianship of a child to age eighteen. Sometimes what begins as foster care ends in adoption. For example, a Christian couple in my community is in the process of adopting their eleven-year-old foster daughter who was recently released for permanent placement. Like the adoption of "special children" foster care is well worth considering but not to be entered into lightly.

The possibilities and pitfalls of foster care, agency versus private adoption, international adoption, and the adoption of hard-to-place children are all subjects on which volumes have been written. Those seriously considering adoption would do well to acquaint themselves with some of the current literature devoted to these subjects (see appendix). *The Adoption Resource Book* by Lois Gilman and *The Adoption Adviser* by Joan McNamara are particularly comprehensive resources. In addition, adoption resource exchanges and adoptive-parent support groups exist in many communities; members readily share information and answer questions.

In the following pages, two questions commonly asked by prospective adoptive parents will be considered: Will I be able to love an adopted child as much as I could love a biological child? And what is the risk that my child will one day search out his or her birth mother? The fear underlying the second question is that a fruitful search might jeopardize the adoptive parent-child relationship.

On Loving "Someone Else's Child"

The story is told of a neighbor who noticed that the parents of an adopted two-year-old stayed overnight in the hospital with her after her tonsillectomy. The neighbor exclaimed, "Why that's just like a *real* mother!"

Adoptive parents are genuinely mystified (and sometimes angered) by such remarks. Teri Yates, who has a biological daughter as well as an adopted daughter, says, "People who ask, 'How can you love someone else's child?' have not reflected on what they're saying. From the minute you receive an adopted child, he or she begins to be yours, not someone else's. There is a parallel with our being adopted into God's kingdom. We're just fortunate that these children are loaned to us for a while to love, cherish, and nurture."

Kathy, who also has both adopted and biological children, agrees: "As common as adoption is, I am amazed that there are still questions about it. We Christians understand that we are all adopted into God's family through Christ's work on the cross. Since we have been adopted by our heavenly Father, adoption should be a logical enough concept for us to grasp. Our adopted son has been such a blessing; it's difficult to imagine our household without him. None of us would be the same!" Teri and Kathy's words are resoundingly affirmed by others.

The delight David and Margaret take in their son Andrew is typical of those who have adopted. Margaret says, "After my doctor told me my chances of getting pregnant were virtually nil, things were much easier for me. I said, 'Okay, if that's the way it is, I can accept it. Let's go ahead with adoption.' I was relieved and happy to know where I was. I no longer had to get depressed every month when I got my period. I said, 'No problem. I know Catholic Charities is there for us.' " Margaret had this assurance because at the beginning of their infertility treatment, she and David put their name in with an adoption agency. They knew from the outset of the infertility workup that their chances of having a biological child were slight, and they also knew the wait for an adopted child was likely to be long. When they called Catholic Charities and asked to be put on their list, they were told to expect a wait of three to four years. By the time their case came up, their infertility had been confirmed.

"Finally, our case study was underway," Margaret recalls, "and I was as nervous as could be, even though I really liked our caseworker. You wonder, 'Are we going to be found worthy to be parents?' I was working in an inner-city school, where I was teaching and loving battered, neglected children. Once I came so close to taking one of those children home with me that, afterward, I got sick thinking about what would have happened to me if I had. I knew the child was neglected, and I loved him so much; I couldn't understand why his mother could have him and I couldn't. So to be put through a parenting test was hard. What the agency was really trying to do was match our background with a baby's, but you don't see it that way when you're going through it. You think, 'Am I good enough? Will I say the wrong thing?' "

Their home study was finished by April, and they were told they would have a baby by the end of the year. But when Margaret was two days into a summer job, they got a call from the agency saying, "We have a baby boy for you. Come pick him up on Thursday at one o'clock." Margaret says, "I floated to Bible study that night and dominated the entire evening with, 'You'll never guess what happened to me today!' Everybody was so happy because everyone had been praying for us. They had been very supportive. One of the women had even gone to the infertility specialist with me on several occasions. They saw to it that by Thursday morning we had a crib, bassinet, a changing table, and two bags of clothes. We had everything anybody would ever need for a baby. All hand-me-downs and all beautiful!

"When we went to pick up our baby, the caseworker began to tell us some sketchy things about his background. All the while, I knew he was in the next room, and I was dying to see him. I said, 'Couldn't we just have a peek?' The caseworker replied, 'Before we go in, I have to tell you that he has a birth defect.' Well, I had an image of a perfect cherub, and I was aghast! The 'defect' turned out to be a tiny bald spot on top of his head, which, to us, didn't matter at all. Finally, we walked into the next room and on a table was a little baby seat, and in the seat was a beautiful baby with a big gummy grin and the hiccups. And he was ours! There was no doubt about it; he was our baby. We just grabbed him. We took him home and the first thing we did was strip him. It was a spontaneous thing. We laid him down and peeled off his clothes as if to say, 'What have we got here?'

"He is now six and an angel. Everybody who knows him loves him. He wants to be a priest, and for two years he has begged the rector to let him be an acolyte. To be an acolyte, Andrew has to be as tall as the candles on the altar, so every three months, we have to measure him to see if he's there yet. He is not perfect by any means, but he is a very loving little boy."

Six months after David and Margaret welcomed their son Andrew into their family, Margaret discovered she was pregnant. At first, the pregnancy was an unwelcome surprise. "I thought I had an ovarian cyst," she says. "It never occurred to me that I might be pregnant. It had been an eleven-year wait, and I had been told by two doctors that I wouldn't get pregnant, and that even if I did, I wouldn't carry the baby to term. So even though I had a perfect pregnancy and never felt or looked better in my life, I never believed I would actually bring the baby home. I didn't even have a bassinet when I went to the hospital.

"I had put being pregnant behind me and didn't even want it any more. I was so happy with Andrew, I didn't want anything to interfere. Also, I found it hard to switch gears. Having to accept the fact that I couldn't have children was easier than finding I was pregnant all of a sudden: 'I'm going to have a baby? But I already have a baby!' Then I went on a guilt trip. There are all these people who want children, I thought, and here I am with one already and about to have another.

"I really don't believe, contrary to the myth, that adopting had anything to do with my getting pregnant. I do believe that all those treatments I had loosened things up enough to finally allow sperm to get through. I think it was a one-shot deal. My biological son, Timothy, is an extremely headstrong child, and I suspect he was in a very determined little sperm that pushed its way through. Actually, being pregnant with Timothy was anticlimactic. I was more fulfilled when I walked out of that adoption agency with Andrew in my arms than I was coming out of the delivery room with Timothy. The one thing I missed with my adopted baby was nursing him. That was the one special difference between adopting and having a biological child.

"God knows the right time for us," Margaret concludes. "He knows our timetable much better than we do. There were many times that seemed right to have a child, but when we actually had our children, the times were right. He knows when we're ready. It *does* work out. You *can* have a child. You can have an adopted child who is as much a part of you—absolutely—as a biological child. I know because I have one of each."

Several of the couples who have contributed to this book have both adopted and biological children, and they all echo Margaret's sentiments. As Kathy says, "Motherhood is much more involved with the actual rearing and nurturing of a child than birthing." Teri Yates agrees. "Twenty-two months after our adopted daughter came to live with us, we were privileged to welcome our second miracle daughter. At last an infertility specialist diagnosed my problem, and our second daughter was conceived. I know the double joy of being a mother through adoption and conception, and I know that mother-child bonding isn't just something that happens at birth. It is a continuous process of daily loving, caring, and touching. I am a mother, not because I gave birth to a baby, but because I function as a mother. I'm the one who dries their tears, applauds their accomplishments, kisses their hurts, and wipes up their messes."

It would be misleading to suggest that every adoption is as idyllic as David's and Margaret's. Snags and delays are common, and some adoptions simply fall through. In private adoptions, the birth mother may have a change of heart, or in the case of foreign adoptions, a country may suddenly be closed due to shifting political winds. As Teri says, "Only the hardy need apply."

Dennis and Nancy know the stress caused by inexplicable delays. An infant girl was assigned to them in mid-August by their agency. It takes an average of three months from the date of assignment for the legal and immigration work to be completed, but at Christmas they were still waiting for their daughter's arrival. Just after Thanksgiving they were informed that the Colombian courts had closed for three weeks and that immigration papers could not be signed until after the New Year.

Winston and Jane, another couple who weathered a bumpy adoption, once wondered if their son, Jeremy, would ever be theirs. Jane says, "From the time we received that phone call from the doctor saying, 'Sorry, there's no hope for you,' I felt like saying, 'Stop the world; I want to get off.' I immediately lost my sense of direction. The prospect of our being without children was the thing that was most disturbing, not that we could not bear children. At the same time we were told we could not bear children, we were also told that adoption was just out of the question.

"The situation looked so bleak. Like most people looking to adopt, I ran the gamut. I did research. I read. I sorted through lists of agencies. Our experience with agencies was pretty depressing. After two years of being wait-listed with one, we were able to take the first step of filling out an application. As the lady from the agency said, 'Business has been bad.' "

The discouraging adoption picture coupled with the pain of their infertility led to stresses in Winston's and Jane's previously stable marriage. Jane says, "Because I lost my certainty about who I was, I was pretty shaken for a couple of years, and we had a lot of ups and downs. During the down times we would say, 'How could we ever bring a child into this rotten relationship? It wouldn't be fair.' Quite often, we felt that it was good to have time to work out problems in our marriage and learn more about each other."

Finally, Jane concluded that her life had been on hold long enough. She began looking for a new job, one that would use her sociology degree. "I wanted to pick my feet up and get them out of the mud they had been stuck in for a couple of years." One day, shortly after she made this resolution, the adoption light turned green.

One afternoon while she was at work, a friend called and casually asked, "What's new? Any children in your life yet?" The caller went on to say that a friend's daughter was pregnant and due in about two weeks. Determined that her daughter give the child up for adoption, the biological grandmother was anxious to place her grandchild in a Christian home. The caller asked Jane to meet the grandmother that afternoon. Jane responded cautiously but she finally agreed to the meeting.

Her conversation with the grandmother launched a complicated chain of events involving lawyers, the birth family, Winston and Jane, and the friends who had originally acted as intermediaries. It quickly became apparent that, while the grandmother was resolute about putting her daughter's baby up for adoption, neither the birth mother or father had made that decision. It took them two months to make up their minds that it was best to give the baby up—two of the most agonizing months in Winston's and Jane's lives. Jane says, "To keep my sanity, I was praying more than I ever had in my life, and it was probably the most selfless praying I've ever done. I remember crying for those grandparents and for those teenage parents who loved each other. It was terribly hard for them to decide to give the baby up. I prayed for them and wept for what they were going through."

"In the end," Jane concludes, "when Jeremy finally became ours, when we got that first phone call saying, 'Yes, he is going to come to you,' I had peace that this indeed was God's will for us. If we had paid an exorbitant fee for a child or used any manipulative ways, I wouldn't have been so at ease. God was there at every step, and I knew that little boy was meant for us." She laughs when she recalls that her initial feelings about adoption were, "I just don't know if I can love an adopted child as much as one we might have produced." It is quite a different picture now. "Today, I know the answer to that question. Jeremy had been in our home for about three days when I said to Winston, 'Oh, how could I have ever thought that I couldn't love this child as much as one born of our own flesh? Jeremy is my little Moses that God put in the bulrushes for me.' "

The Search for Biological Roots

In addition to wondering if they could love an adopted child as much as they could love a "natural" child, prospective adoptive parents are often apprehensive about the possibility that one day their child might search out his or her biological roots. They fear rejection and wonder if the investment of many years could suddenly be undermined by the appearance of the birth mother. The specter of the search is not to be taken lightly, but it is seldom a calamitous event.

To begin with, very few couples today are secretive about their child's adopted status. In fact, most make a virtue of it. As Janet, the mother of two, says, "The Word often speaks about the privilege of being adopted into God's family, and we want our children to know that to be adopted is special, that they were chosen. There's a chorus that goes: 'Praise the Lord, I'm adopted in the family. Praise the Lord, I'm a child of the King.' We sing this with our children daily, putting their names into the song to make it more personal." Margaret says, "We forget Andrew's adopted and so do his grandparents. It's not in the forefront of our thinking, and yet it's not hidden either. Andrew has always known he is adopted. We have read *The Chosen Baby* to him, and I would often say, when I put him to bed at night, 'I'm so glad we adopted you. That was the best thing we ever did.' One time, when I was kissing him good-night, he said, 'I'm so glad I adopted you, Mommy!' Every once in a while he asks a question about adoption, which we answer without elaboration. We tell our sons, 'God gave both of you to us. He just gave you to us in different ways.' "

Such openness lays the groundwork for answering the serious questions that may arise later in childhood or adolescence. Typical of many, Margaret says, "I don't know how I'll handle it if and when Andrew becomes interested in finding his birth mother. How do I know how I will react? I do know how Andrew feels about us, however; and if, when he is of age, he wants to seek out his biological mother, I will certainly help him do it. It would be an awfully hard thing to go through, but I know where I stand with him."

While most adopted children have a normal curiosity about their birth parents, a minority actually search for them. Should a child decide to search, there is no guarantee of success. Despite a trend toward "open adoptions," in which the adoptive and birth families know each other's identities, the adoption process is still generally shrouded in a secrecy that some adoptees resent. Records are closed in most states, and a court order is required to open them. In England, where adoption records were recently opened, fewer than one percent of all adoptees are searching for their birth parents. In the United States, there are considerable legal obstacles to a successful search.

Yet for most adoptees, a reluctance to hurt their adoptive parents is a more compelling reason for hesitating to investigate their genetic heritage. The majority of adoptees who do look for their biological parents are females. Most are much more interested in finding their birth mothers than they are in locating their birth fathers, and many postpone the search until they marry and have children of their own.

While it is risky to generalize about the motivation of those who search or the effects of the search on the adoptive family, I believe the following accounts are fairly representative. Lee, the adoptive daughter of Jack and Phyllis, loves her parents and has always had a good relationship with them. Yet she struggled in adolescence with feelings of "I'm a nobody." In her case, the usual problems of adolescence were aggravated by a sense that because she was adopted, a piece of her identity was missing. One day she discovered her adoption papers in a drawer along with her birth certificate. Finding those papers, which bore her birth mother's last name, marked the beginning of her search.

However, it was not until her twenty-seventh birthday that she actually met her birth mother. Reluctant to risk hurting her parents and afraid of their rejection, she repeatedly postponed her investigation. However, when her first and second pregnancies were complicated by medical problems, she was prompted to learn more about her medical history. With relative ease, she found both her birth mother and birth father. The result? Although her contact with them has been slight, Lee says, "I feel for the first time that I have no skeletons in my closet, and I'm much more stable emotionally. That 'black hole,' that piece of my identity that was missing, has been found."

It took Lee a year and a half to find the courage to tell Jack and Phyllis—the people she has never stopped seeing as her parents—that she had located her birth mother and father. Then one night, while she and her husband were visiting her parents, she began, haltingly, to tell them what she had done. Jack's response was characteristically calm. "Well, it really doesn't matter, because regardless of what your relationship is with them now, they can never take away what we've had. You will always be ours."

Phyllis responded differently. Once Lee's announcement sank in, she felt rejected. "The following week was black. I'm just thankful I had my granddaughter with me to mother all week. When I took her home the next week, I had a list of questions for Lee." Phyllis agonized that something she had done or neglected to do during Lee's upbringing had prompted the search, but Lee quickly put her fears to rest. She said, "Mother, it wasn't anything you did or didn't do. The only way I can describe it is that my life was like a pie with a piece missing. Now, it's whole."

Lee observes that during the eighteen months she waited to tell her parents about the search, their relationship had not suffered. In fact, Lee believes that it had actually improved, since she no longer had unanswered questions. Today Phyllis and Jack enjoy a sound and loving relationship with their daughter, and they dote on the two grandchildren she has given them.

Mary Jane, another adoptee who searched for her birth mother, also has reassuring words for those considering adoption: "When I began to search at age forty-nine, I was looking for ethnic and biological information. I was curious about where my forebears had come from and why I looked the way I did. Also, I had some curiosity about why one of my children was born with a Mongolian spot, a little blue birthmark that appears at the base of a baby's spine and goes away after about three months. When I took an anthropology course as an adult college student, I learned that a Mongolian spot is a racial characteristic limited to just a few groups—bushmen in Africa, Mongolians, American Indians, and as I later learned, some Mediterranean Jews. My daughter and I used to play at making up ancestors. We made up Indian princesses, and Genghis Khan, and all kinds of interesting people. Another factor in my search was that I had some medical difficulties in adulthood, and it became more important to learn about my biological inheritance. I just needed to fill in the blanks. I had wonderful parents, and I think of those who adopted and raised me so carefully and lovingly as my mother and father. God was so gracious to me, and I was very fortunate in that home.

"When I contacted the agency through which I was adopted and learned I had a sister, I was seized with the need to find her and learn if she was all right. She has since become a very dear friend, and we enjoy having her six children, our nieces and nephews, as part of our lives. I also became anxious to meet my birth mother and tell her how well life had treated me and how fortunate I had been. I wanted her to know what a good decision she had made and how thankful I was that she had the courage to allow me to be placed in a home that had given me so many advantages.

"I did have the chance to meet her and thank her before she died, and I learned some interesting information. She described to me an absolutely disastrous family system—a system of marriages that were easily left and of children who were, perhaps not easily, but willingly given to others to raise when the going got tough. A system perpetuated by a daughter she later adopted and raised. I became convinced that I was rescued from that family system. There is no reason to think that my life would have followed a different pattern if I had been raised by her. Instead, I was raised in a family of deep Christian faith and deep commitment to values, morals, and family strength. I'm really thankful for that."

There are no guarantees for adoptive parents any more than there are for parents generally, and the road to adoption can be hard and full of unexpected turns. Nevertheless, adoption remains a wonderful alternative for those who long to include a child in their lives. As one adoptive mother says, "The wait, the cost, and even the infertility are worth it!"

Because I Was Adopted
by Teri Yates[1]

a tribute to my parents
who chose to adopt
a little three-year- old Amerasian girl
with rotten baby teeth, bloated stomach, and infected ears,
and call me their own

Because I was adopted
    I knew I was chosen, I was wanted.
Because I was adopted
    I no longer know hunger, the pain of discrimination,
        the lack of a land to call my own.
Because I was adopted
    I had plenty of food to eat and clothes to wear.
Because I was adopted
    I know that love is unconditional.
Because I was adopted
    I attended private schools
        and received a college education.
Because I was adopted
    I know the love of parents who pray for me daily.
Because I was adopted
    I know the love of a husband and
        I have children to nurture.
Because I was adopted
    I know who I am. I'm me, unique,
        special, created by God.
Because I was adopted
    I feel every child deserves a permanent home.

Because I was adopted
    I am stronger in spirit and
        challenged to appreciate and
    care about my fellow man whatever handicaps
        he may have—
emotional, physical, or spiritual.
Because I was adopted
    I believe in God. He has kept me
        in the palm of His hand.

–8–

Desert Flowers

REGARDLESS OF HOW INFERTILITY IS RESOLVED—BY PREGNANCY, adoption, or deciding to remain childless—infertility need not be merely an unproductive hiatus in one's life, a desert where nothing flowers. One of the great things about the Christian faith is that it gives us a framework for disarming pain and suffering, for turning it to constructive, rather than destructive ends.

In the healing of my own grief, I found this instruction from the letter of James helpful: "When all kinds of trials and temptations crowd into your lives . . . don't resent them as intruders but welcome them as friends! Realize that they come to test your faith and to produce in you the quality of endurance" (James 1:2-3, PHILLIPS). These words from 2 Corinthians have also been encouraging: "Thank God, the Father of our Lord Jesus Christ, that he is our Father and the source of all mercy and comfort. For he gives us comfort in our trials so that we in turn may be able to give the same sort of strong sympathy to others in theirs" (2 Corinthians 1:3-4, PHILLIPS).

What these verses say to me is that nothing need be wasted in the Christian life. No experience, however bleak or painful, need be written off as an exercise in futility. Childlessness, like other disappointments, can easily lead to bitterness and self-pity or, by the grace of God, can result in greater self-knowledge, a stronger, more mature faith, and a larger capacity for compassion for others. Even in the midst of our barrenness, God can bring forth life.

Compassion

Growth in compassion is one of the most unmistakable common denominators among infertile Christians. Typical of many are Tracy's remarks: "I can now truly thank God for this whole infertility experience. It has made both my husband and me more compassionate when dealing with the trials and heartaches experienced by members of our church, and it has also made us more sensitive to hurting people in all walks of life. I thank God for this season of weeping, for how could I ever fully taste and appreciate the joys of life without first passing through the bitter waters of sorrow?" Indeed, there is nothing quite so effective as pain in alerting us to the sorrows and needs of others.

When I asked Marjory Bankson if she had any misgivings about deciding not to become a mother, she replied, "I have some sadness. Each of my sisters has an eldest child who looks like me, and there are times, particularly when I am with those two girls, that I am very sad that they are not my children.

"Yet it seems to me," Marjory continued, "that the regrets that I have help keep me in touch with the reality of my life. I live a terrifyingly comfortable life, and my middle-class affluence is dangerous because it can remove me from my bondedness to other members of God's creation. It's terribly easy for me to stay in my house or at my job and send out lots of letters and be in a rather abstract communication with other people of my kind.

"So the pain in my life is really a gift. It's the pain that allows me to take in my stray sheep when they come. It's the pain in my life that allows me to respond to my widowed neighbor who drinks too much and is really an annoying person to be with. I look at her, and I imagine myself alone and afraid and perhaps afflicted with the glaucoma that plagues her life, and it gives me the patience to take her to the doctor or read her a newspaper article or listen one more time when she calls and needs to talk.

"It's the pain in my life that alerts me to how common I am and reminds me of my bondedness to others. So I wouldn't do without it. I wouldn't have it miraculously wiped out. I believe we each are given an allotment of difficulties and joys, and our spiritual journey is largely the working out of how to love in the middle of that—how to love myself, how to love those close at hand, and how to love those in an increasingly larger circle."

Marjory's words ring true to me. One clear fall afternoon when I was in the hospital for my ruptured appendix, I had a flash of insight. I was awake, lucid, and snug in my hospital bed despite the constant intravenous drip of antibiotics and the quiet rattle of the nasal-gastric tube taped above my lip. The sun was streaming through the large picture window by my bed. Lying there, looking out over the fields below and enjoying the warmth of the sunlight, I suddenly saw myself suspended above the earth with an astronaut's perspective on the oceans and continents below. From that vantage point, held but a moment, I looked into lands where there were masses of poorly clad, homeless, hungry, and diseased people. Despite their numbers, I saw not faceless hordes but individuals.

In that brief instant I saw, with perfect clarity, that any pain, loss, or misfortune that I had known or would ever know was but a tiny drop in the flood of affliction that is the common lot of mankind. This realization, so basic that it embarrasses me to call it an "insight," did not depress me. Rather, I felt strangely comforted and warmed. Lying there in my own minor distress, I felt kinship with all who suffer and more a part of the human family than I had ever felt before. This momentary glimpse into my bondedness to others left its mark.

Months later, when my doctor informed me of my infertility and told me my tubes were terribly scarred, even "clubbed," I felt blighted and ashamed at first. But when I recalled the picture given to me in the hospital, my shock at being crippled, even in a hidden organ, was transformed. Instead of shrinking from my disability, I began to see it as a small but significant point of contact with others whose bodies were bent or broken. Not only could I more clearly identify with those who were broken in body, I could also better understand those who mourned or were poor in spirit.

I began to see that the sorrow of childlessness like any other sorrow can lead us out from the shallows of complacency and self-sufficiency to deeper places of caring and humility. Like most people, I would rather wear the emblems of "success" than the marks of suffering. Yet I also know that even Jesus, who became like us in every respect to bring us to salvation, became perfect through suffering. I began to see that just as his redemptive suffering provides the means of reconciliation between God and mankind, our pain can break down the artificial barriers we erect between ourselves and others, and bond us to them in shared humanity. Rather than isolating us, our infertility can become a bridge to others who are hurting.

Often where there is the greatest theological orthodoxy, there is the least love and compassion. If, in response to the comfort the Lord gives us in our sorrow, we become more compassionate people, we will bear a gift that the Church and the world sorely need. In addition to increasing our capacity for compassion, the sorrow of infertility can also act as a refiner's fire, strengthening and purifying our faith.

Why Me, Lord?

This morning I rummaged in a desk drawer to find a small book, boxed and wrapped in tissue paper for safekeeping, its white cover stamped "Marriage Service" in gold script. Paging through the thin volume, I came to the neatly typed insert containing the personal remarks the minister addressed to my husband and me on our wedding day. The comments of our brother-in-law David, the Presbyterian clergyman who married us, were based on a text we had selected: "I will give them one heart and one way, that they may fear Me always, for their own good, and for the good of their children after them" (Jeremiah 32:39, NASB).

When I came upon that verse in my devotional reading years ago, it struck me as apt for our wedding because it reflected my view of marriage as a relationship blessed by and dependent upon God, a relationship into which children would eventually come and receive his blessing also. Years later, when I found I was infertile, this verse that I had "claimed" puzzled me. Had I misunderstood? Had I heard wrong? Like the majority of involuntarily childless Christians, I sought to understand my infertility not as an isolated issue but within the context of my faith in God.

Today I look back with affection and some amusement at the twenty-one-year-old who blithely appropriated for herself a promise given to the nation of Israel, a promise that *could* apply to individuals but which, in its context, has nothing to do with marriage between two people. I have since realized that such casual and misguided handling of Scripture, however sincere, can lead to unnecessary confusion and sometimes cause real pain. For instance, one earnest couple read a book that claimed Scripture as its authority, a book that hinted that pregnancy would follow a step of faith like buying diapers; they went one better and bought a crib. "At first it was exciting, and we rejoiced and prayed over it," the wife recalls, "but after a while I began to feel the crib was a threat from my husband—'I purchased this; now you do your part and fill it.' I would never suggest that anyone else do something like that. It hurt too much to see that crib standing empty."

Infertile Christians turn to the Scriptures for guidance and illumination, and there is great consolation and strength to be found there. However, it is very important to read and interpret the Bible with care. As Rosemarie Manganello and Linda Anderson observe, the Old Testament blessings and curses concerning barrenness must be understood in their cultural setting. It would have been far more difficult to be infertile in a patriarchal age, such as the Old Testament era, when children were of great economic importance and a woman's worth lay almost entirely in her ability to bear them. A barren woman, like a barren field, was useless. If one looks to a different era, to the New Testament teachings of Jesus Christ, there is not the slightest hint of such an attitude. Manganello and Anderson also note that promises such as "Delight yourself in the Lord, and he will give you the desires of your heart" must not be lifted out of context and narrowly applied to this one dimension of our lives.[1]

The Bible is not a magic book containing incantations to ward off infertility or make it disappear. Nor does the Bible provide neat and tidy answers to the mystery and pain of barrenness. Even for theologians the "why" of infertility is elusive. Timothy Weber, associate professor of church history at Denver Conservative Baptist Seminary, describes how he and his wife Linda wrestled with their infertility. In an *Eternity* article entitled "Empty Quivers," he writes, "We are Christians, so we were never alone in our struggles. But in some ways, being believers made things *worse*, not better. The God we believe in is not a disinterested bystander who is unmoved by the needs and suffering of his people. He cares for them. He even intervenes to save them and relieve their pain.

"We read the Bible and found that it contains numerous stories of 'barren women' for whom God had provided children—Sarah and Rachel in Genesis, the wife of Manoah in Judges, Hannah in 1 Samuel, and Elizabeth in the Gospel of Luke. We discovered Psalm 113 and thought it spoke directly to our need: 'The Lord is exalted over all the nations, his glory above the heavens. Who is like the Lord our God, the One who sits enthroned on high, who stoops down to look on the heavens and the earth? He raises the poor from the dust and lifts the needy from the ash heap; he seats them with princes, with the princes of their people. He settles the barren woman in her home as a happy mother of children' (Psalm 113:4-9).

"God had given children to them. Why not us? For Linda and me—and many other infertile Christian couples—a medical problem turned into a spiritual crisis.

"By far the most difficult part of our struggle centered on our inability to figure out why God had allowed our infertility problem. We came up with elaborate theories. Of course, being a seminary professor did not help matters. I was supposed to have all the answers; but it soon became apparent that I did not. . . . Finally we stopped trying to determine God's reasons. He has his own purposes but never let us in on them.

"God became more personal—and much more mysterious. His actions became difficult to understand, more inscrutable. We no longer viewed him as a cosmic vending machine that delivered whatever we selected from its storehouse of goodies or as a doting father who bestowed on his children whatever their hearts desired. We were forced to trust God, even when his actions . . . were incomprehensible to us.

"In short, we got used to living on God's terms, not ours. It was a terribly difficult lesson to learn. It is never easy to put your life in God's hands, especially when you believe that he is not going to give you what you want. After nearly six years, we found we could think positively about the future, take our lives off "hold," and be happy again. We learned to be thankful for what we had—each other, our health, important work to do, and a God who really cares for us—and not to dwell on what we did not have."

The Webers' story does not end there. To their great joy, six months after a "final surgery," Linda became pregnant, and today they have not one but two children. Timothy concludes, "We still do not know why we had to go through all that we did, but we are changed people because of it. Though it has been nearly two years since our infertility ended . . . we are unable to put (it) completely behind us. It is one of those traumas that people never really get over. But we can be encouraging to people who have a similar problem, and not just because we ended up having the family that we so desperately wanted. We found hope and even a sense of peace *during* our struggle, and learned how to be joyful *despite* our infertility. Thanks to the grace of God, we found that our 'quiver' *was* full, whether we had children or not."[2]

The Silences of God

Like Timothy Weber, May, a former teacher from Michigan, found that "in some respects, being a Christian made infertility more difficult. Why was God choosing not to bless our union with a child? Had we sinned in some way? I became adept at picking out the condemnatory passages of

Scripture and deciding that they applied to me. My earthly father has always been cold, distant, and impossible to please, and that is exactly how God appeared to me.

"God let me rant and rave until I was ready to be quiet, and I'm thankful he is so patient. Even though some Christians reacted to our dilemma with clichés such as, 'If God seems distant, guess who moved,' I finally realized the spiritual desert and the silences of God are legitimate experiences backed up in Scripture. The only thing that kept me going was walking by faith, going back to God's Word, and saying, 'Your Word says that you love me. Even though I don't feel it and things don't look like it to me, I will believe it.' "

May, who is now thirty-nine, and her husband Gary, an optometrist in his early forties, recently resolved what they call their "third experience with infertility." Their particular journey has been long and marked with heartbreaking turns, turns that have tried but not shattered their resilient faith. After nearly six years of marriage, May gave birth to their first child. "We settled into parenthood like ducks to water," she recollects, "I loved every minute of it. I didn't even mind the colic and the dirty diapers."

When their son David was one-and-a-half, May and Gary began to hope for a second child, but only after about eighteen months of trying to conceive did May become pregnant again. "That pregnancy did not go well," she remembers. "I had funny feelings of dread, or premonition, that something was very wrong." After a difficult delivery, their second child, Katie, was born, and it soon became apparent that she had serious birth defects. Specialists diagnosed a congenital syndrome that could cause epilepsy, mental retardation, and cerebral palsy. However, the doctors could not say with any certainty what Katie's eventual condition might be. May and Gary could only wait.

"After hearing the doctor's diagnosis," May says, "I went home and went through at least six of the most horrible months of my life. The infertility was part of it—becoming pregnant had been such a long difficult process. At length, I was able to realize that God plans each life, as he says in Psalm 139, well before the moment of conception. He knows exactly what each child will be like. He had Katie's life planned perhaps since the foundation of the world, and he had sent her for his own purposes that were not mine to question. So I asked his forgiveness for what was essentially rebellion in not wanting to raise a handicapped child, and I turned my whole life over to him.

"It was amazing how quickly my feelings and attitudes changed and my grief and depression lifted. Katie became a tremendous joy and blessing to me, although of course I would have loved for her to have been healthy and able to learn and do all the things I wanted for her. God did such fantastic things through Katie. She became his little messenger who shared his love with us, transforming our family and changing us into different and much better people. She touched so many lives around her even though she could never walk or talk at all." Like the Webers, May and Gary experienced the redemptive power of suffering and learned to trust God and affirm his love despite their circumstances.

Katie lived to be almost four years old. Born when May was thirty-one, she died quite suddenly when May was thirty-five. From the time Katie was a year old, May sorely wanted another child, and nearly three years after Katie died, May conceived again. "I was always going to have my family complete by age thirty-five," May says. "No way was I going to run the higher risks of birth defects by trying to have children after thirty-five. But here I am about to give birth at age thirty-nine and very happy about it. Will this child I am carrying be normal? Only God knows for sure. Regardless, it is a life planned by him for his good purpose, a purpose I am committed to helping him carry out."

I am delighted to report that May has since given birth to Amy Janna, a healthy eight-pound, fourteen-ounce girl, whose name means "beloved gift of God." Printed on the pink announcement of her birth were these words: "O Lord, I will honor and praise your name, for You are my God; You do such wonderful things!" (Isaiah 25:1, TLB).

On Being Blessed

As we have seen, not all infertility is resolved by pregnancy, and standing by and watching others have their first, second, or third child can be deeply troubling for those who are earnestly praying for children. A California woman writes, "After eight months of trying to conceive her second child, a friend asked for prayer from her women's group and went forward at a healing service. A month later, she was pregnant. We, too, have sought prayer for years and have gone forward at a healing service. It hurts not to know why our prayers for a child have not been answered."

One reason unanswered prayer for children is puzzling is that so many pregnancies are unwanted. More than 3,000,000 unintended pregnancies occur in the United States annually.[3] Approximately fifty percent of these mistimed or undesired pregnancies end in abortion. Moreover, UNICEF figures indicate that *every day* more than 40,000 of the world's children die—a truly horrifying statistic that should prompt us all to personal and political action to end world hunger. In some quarters, life seems so cheap. In others, it seems so maddeningly elusive.

There are no easy answers to this puzzle. Yet the "why" of infertility is not really the ultimate question; nor is whether or not we have children of ultimate importance. More important is whether we turn from God in the midst of our barrenness or go on trusting him, even when we are convinced that what we desire most will not be given us. While the reason for our infertility will very likely remain a mystery, I believe that if we offer our barrenness to God, he will always bring forth life. But life, as Timothy Weber says, "on his terms." We may go on to bear children. We may adopt them. Or we may remain childless. Regardless, we are called to seek God, serve him, and find his blessing in the present.

Among the passages of Scripture infertile Christians find most disconcerting is "Sons are a heritage from the Lord, children a reward from him. Like arrows in the hands of a warrior are sons born in one's youth. Blessed is the man whose quiver is full of them" (Psalm 127:3-5). Manganello and Anderson note that such passages can cause needless anguish unless we see that children are among God's many gifts—they come to us as a result of God's grace rather than because we are deserving.[4]

Many who have contributed to this book agree. In recalling the birth of her first child, a birth that came only after years of waiting and repeated miscarriages, Kathy says, "Our son's birth made us appreciate all the gifts the good Lord has given us, gifts we had tended to forget. The gift of marriage. Our salvation in Christ. There were many gifts we had undervalued. We began to see life as a whole series of gifts and to realize that to dwell on the one gift of children is limiting."

In a remarkable passage in the Gospel of Luke (Luke 11:27-28), Jesus is teaching, and a woman in the crowd calls out, "Blessed is the mother who gave you birth and nursed you." Here, if ever there was one, was a golden opportunity for Jesus to give a homily on the ultimate blessedness of motherhood and the biological family. Instead, he replies, "Blessed rather are those who hear the word of God and obey it." Jesus clearly values the family and loved his own. Even as he was dying on the Cross, he provided for his mother, commending her and his disciple John to each other's care. But Jesus was not sentimental about biological relationships, nor did he ever proclaim family or children the ultimate reality or good. He says blessed *rather* are those who seek his face. Blessed *rather* are those who seek to discern his purpose for their lives. Blessed *rather* are those who participate in the building of his eternal kingdom. That is his word to each of us, regardless of whether or not we have children.

To me, though we catch just a glimpse of her, one of the great figures in the Bible is Anna the prophetess. When I think of the Bible and barrenness, I think of her as well as figures like Sarah, Hannah, and Elizabeth. A dependent of the temple, Anna was not only widowed but apparently childless as well. She was therefore in a precarious position.

Titus Presler, an Episcopal priest who is presently a missionary to Africa, comments on the position of women like Anna in biblical times: "In the time of Jesus, widows were among the most vulnerable and unprotected people of Israel, and so they were among the most deprived and oppressed. Livelihoods were available mainly to men. When a woman's husband died, her rights of inheritance were very limited. When a woman had a son, she had to depend on him. If she had no children, she could return to her parents. Otherwise, her best bet was to marry her husband's brother. Failing all of this she was fully exposed: There was no Social Security, no pension, no benefits to collect, no life insurance. She had no rights, and she was prey to unscrupulous lawyers, humiliation, and finally, poverty. The prophecies of Scripture often rail against this oppression."[5]

In spite of her vulnerability and precarious circumstances, we find Anna devoted to service in the house of the God. When Joseph and Mary took the infant Jesus to the temple to be circumcised, Anna was there. In the Gospel of Luke we find this capsule description of her: "She was very old; she had lived with her husband seven years after her marriage, and then was a widow until she was eighty-four. She never left the temple but worshiped night and day, fasting and praying." Coming up to Joseph and Mary and the baby Jesus, Anna "gave thanks to God and spoke about the child to all who were looking forward to the redemption of Jerusalem" (Luke 2:36-38).

Without husband, without family, without even one child—Anna stood alone at the crossroads of history, pointing men and women in the direction of God. Despite her personal circumstances, she was rich in spirit and content in her heart.

Anna lost herself in the worship and service of God. And into the poverty of her life, Jesus came.

Afterthoughts

I was twenty-seven years old when I had the ruptured appendix that put an end to our expectations of having children of "our own." A few years later, when I wrote the first edition of *Without Child*, I was thirty-four. On my last birthday, I hit the milestone of forty. At each of these three stages, my experience of infertility, and the issues it raises, has been somewhat different.

Those early years of discovering and coming to terms with our childlessness were undoubtedly the most difficult in some respects. For one thing, the pain was fresh and therefore sharp. For another, the years when my husband and I were in our mid- and late twenties were, quite naturally, the ones when many of our friends were having their babies. As a result, we felt a bit isolated and out of the mainstream. Also, my own sense of identity was still fragile. I had imagined I would be the mother of several children and that their care would be my principal vocation, at least for a number of years. Coming to see my life in different terms took some time.

Later, when I was in my early and mid-thirties and busy as an executive assistant to the president of Gordon College, a Christian liberal arts college here in Massachusetts, I found my infertility far less painful than it had been initially. In fact, I sometimes felt like mine was the best of all possible worlds. I had the companionship of a loving husband, work that gave me a sense of purpose, and a modest measure of financial freedom, which enabled us not only to travel widely—our chief luxury—but to act out of choice rather than necessity in several areas of my life. For example, I had the liberty of taking a year off from paid employment to write *Without Child*.

During the last few years, the years preceding my fortieth birthday, infertility has become less serious in some respects and more serious in others. The days of being regularly invited to baby showers have long since passed, and the world of young mothers—of diapering and feeding infants, pushing baby strollers, and making visits to the pediatrician— seems quite remote. Today, many of our closest friends' children are learning to drive and beginning to fill out applications to college, while their parents are trying to figure out how to foot the bills. At this point, neither my husband, who is forty-three, nor I have the slightest interest in having a baby.

In one of the ironies familiar to those who are infertile, my husband's twin sister, Penny, who thought her family was complete, had a "surprise" baby at forty-one. That pregnancy required a major adjustment for her; and, during the nine months of learning to accept the unexpected, she occasionally had fantasies about handing the baby off to us. We would have hastily passed him back, because, while we think our nephew Jeffrey is a delightful little fellow, we do not at all envy Penny's having to keep pace with a tireless toddler.

Nor do I envy the young women I meet in the corporate world where I sometimes work on a contract, or temporary, basis. For many of these women, the work day begins at around six-thirty in the morning with a commute in heavy traffic and ends after seven in the evening, when they must set about making dinner and keeping their households going. They seem to be running from one end of their lives to the other. When their children arrive, they take the few weeks of maternity leave available to them, and then they come back to jobs they must keep if they are to make their mortgage payments and pay their other bills. Most of these young women are not trying to "have it all"; they and their husbands are simply trying to make it in difficult economic times. Sooner or later, there will be a backlash against this consuming two-career "lifestyle," which, for many, is really not much of a life at all. When enough people start saying "enough already," some creative alternatives to this model will be found.

Incidentally, as I talk with couples considering adoption, financial concerns seem to loom larger and larger. For instance, a reader from

Minnesota called me several months ago. Her husband had been laid off from his job for some time and had only recently returned to work. Already saddled with debt, they couldn't see how they could afford the several thousand dollars it would cost them to adopt a child. In addition, they were in their late thirties and becoming increasingly comfortable with remaining childless. They simply didn't know how to respond to the other couples in their support group who insisted they "would be sorry" if they didn't adopt.

This woman called me partly to ask me if she and her husband could know, with certainty, which way they should go. Of course, I couldn't answer that question for her. I could only respond that I believe we can trust the desires of our hearts, and if theirs weren't inclining them toward adoption, then they could depend on the Lord to lead them in some other fruitful direction. "But how," the woman insisted, "can we know for certain?" Again, I had no easy answer. I replied that while she and her husband could certainly pray for clarity on this issue, the Lord has given us the power and freedom of choice. No edict was going to be handed down to them from heaven; they would have to accept the responsibility of deciding. And if they decided to remain without children, they could count on living with a certain amount of ambivalence. For obvious reasons, there are more "what ifs" for those who remain childless than there are for the great majority whose infertility is medically resolved or resolved through adoption.

From time to time, my husband and I have felt some of that ambivalence, have raised some of those "what ifs." Until you reach an age where adoption is no longer feasible, the issue of whether or not to adopt is never entirely closed. For us, however, those nagging little questions became less and less significant. We continue to affirm adoption as a wonderful alternative, but I continue to believe the healthiest choices in favor of adoption are made by those who, like Margaret in chapter two, want to have a child not to conform, or feel complete, or prove themselves but "to meet a need to have someone to care for, someone to take the overflow of (their) love." It's a choice best made freely and not out of a panicky sense of necessity.

For us the adoption issue is now closed, and, at this stage of our lives, we are greatly enjoying our freedom and the opportunities it offers us. For example, when my husband was on sabbatical last year, we spent the winter volunteering our time at a Christian college in Kenya, East Africa. He taught two sections of mathematics and pursued a research project, and I edited several college publications. We were also able to travel in Kenya and Tanzania and enjoy the spectacular landscape and wildlife there. Having children would certainly not have automatically precluded our making such a journey; after all, many missionaries and other expatriate families travel and live in places more remote and primitive than Kenya. Yet, since we went on this short-term mission at our own expense, the cost of including children would have been not just daunting for us but probably prohibitive. This trip, one of the most rewarding experiences of our lives, is a good example of the sort of risk we would be far less likely to take if we had children and had to be concerned about providing for their futures.

While we enjoy our freedom and find that the desire for a baby is, for the most part, only a memory, we both have an increasing need for feeling connected with others. Although we can look to each other for warmth and intimacy and affection, we are aware that no marriage can bear the burden of being all things to both partners. To meet our need for community, for feeling linked to others in significant ways, we must reach beyond each other and beyond our biological families.

I grew up in Miami, Florida, at a time when that city lacked its present glamour and notoriety. Yet, when I was in junior and senior high school, the drugs which keep Miami in the national news were already widely available. Both of my troubled younger brothers, who had very slender moorings and who were deeply involved in drug use, committed suicide within six months of each other. I was then twenty-three.

I have no other brothers or sisters, nor are there extended family members who have ever played more than an incidental part in my life. The loss of my brothers, coupled with my inability to bear children, has resulted in being cut off from family in a couple of different directions. As I get older, and particularly as my parents age, I feel the significance of that more and more. I know there will soon come a time when my biological family is history. Moreover, my husband's family is small and geographically distant. There is some sadness for us in these facts, but we don't feel particularly gloomy or morbid about them. Rather, they simply underscore the need for us to work at building significant relationships with others.

Our friends have always been important to us, but, in the future, I think it will become increasingly necessary for us to build an intentional family, a community of Christian friends with whom we can share our love and our lives. For the last few years, several of our closest friends have been single people near our age, some divorced and some never married, who share one or two of our interests and who seem to find our home a comfortable place to be. Their ability to pick up and go with little notice makes it easy for us to be part of each other's social lives.

We also belong to a Bible study of some fourteen or sixteen members, married and single, with children and without, from thirty-something to seventy-plus. We meet twice a month, year after year, to work through various books of the Bible and share prayer concerns. We also laugh a good deal when we're together, and we throw a veritable feast of a potluck dinner several times a year. The fellowship of these friends becomes richer and more valued with the passage of time and the accumulation of shared experiences.

We are, after all, made to live in relationship. The life of God, which was made manifest on this earth in his son Jesus Christ, is lived out and finds its meaning within the fellowship of believers. It is a life meant to be shared—not merely within the narrow confines of the nuclear family but within the larger context of the body of believers. As someone has said, "It's not just Jesus and me; it's Jesus and we."

Until recently, I was having a hard time feeling connected in our large, rather formal liturgical church. When I accepted the responsibility of teaching an adult education series, I found the church a more receptive place than it had previously seemed. Getting involved was the key. I want to continue to take a number of small steps such as that one in order to extend my acquaintance there. I also want to help my husband do the same by more regularly entertaining others in our home.

Just as being childless creates a need to reach out to others beyond my small family circle, it also continues to affect my vocational choices. After nearly ten years in college administration, I realized it was time for a change. While there were things about my work I liked and which gave me a sense of accomplishment, I found myself wishing for more direct involvement with individuals and their needs. The psychologist Erik Erikson talks about a stage of individual development called "generativity" in which we become strongly motivated to contribute to others' growth; perhaps that is part of what is operating in my life now.

For years, I have been sought out by friends and acquaintances in crises of one kind or another. Listening and being a lay counselor of sorts has been a second calling running parallel to the other work I've been doing. In many ways, listening to others relate their troubles and trying to respond constructively has been the most satisfying work I've done. Yet I've never been under any illusion about how complicated our family and personal problems can be. Recognizing the narrow limits of my knowledge and experience, I have referred a number of people to professional therapists. Now I want to come out of my counseling "closet" and obtain the tools I need to become a professional therapist myself; later this year, I will begin a graduate program toward becoming a licensed counselor in private practice.

The absence of children in my life gives me the freedom to return to graduate school as well as the impetus to find meaningful and creative ways to invest in the lives of others. The prospect of preparing for this new vocation at a time when life had gone a bit flat has given me a fresh sense of adventure, for which I am grateful.

There are still moments when I feel the ache of having "empty arms" and the alienation of being on the outside looking in. In Kenneth Grahame's *Wind in the Willows*, one of my favorite children's books, Rat and Mole are lost and far from home on a wintry night. Stopping on their way through a village to peer into glowing cottage windows, they find scenes of warm, cheery, firelit domesticity, before an icy rain sends them scurrying on their way. When I'm feeling a bit sentimental, I'm tempted to think that this is a true picture of the world—that somewhere "out there" the majority are living in cozy domestic bliss. When I start woolgathering in this way, I have to remind myself quickly that this perspective is nine-tenths illusion.

We live in a society where nontraditional households will soon outnumber traditional ones and where millions live lives of lonely desperation. Furthermore, traditional families, which we love to idealize, have plenty of struggles of their own. No one's life is exempt from pain.

As M. Scott Peck so bluntly puts it: "Life is difficult." This short statement is the first sentence in *The Road Less Traveled*, a book about spiritual growth that has been on *The New York Times'* best-seller list for an unprecedented number of weeks. With one part of our minds, we know that Peck, a Christian psychiatrist, is right: Life *is* difficult. Yet, being great escape artists, we want to deny this hard truth. Our almost instinctive reaction to trouble of any kind is fearful or angry surprise: How can this be happening to me? Infertility is but one example of this. As we have seen, those who experience it know the shock and disbelief that come with discovery.

Infertility, like life in general, is undeniably difficult. It, too, presents us with a series of problems and challenges that we can ignore, simply complain about, or seek to resolve. In my own experience, the process of coming to terms with the challenges presented by infertility is ongoing. I think I have this issue resolved once and for all, and then some new dimension of it comes to light or some familiar aspect takes on new meaning. I wouldn't have chosen this path for myself, yet finding myself on it, I see that being childless continues to offer opportunities for change and growth. Like the good that can come out of other forms of suffering, however, the good that may come out of our infertility is good out of evil. For infertility is but one symptom of the brokenness of this fallen world.

Christianity does not ask us to deny the painful reality of evil and suffering on this fractured planet. We are Christians, not stoics. Ours is not the religion of the stiff upper lip. Nowhere in the Bible does it say, "When the going gets tough, the tough get going." Too often we think that Christianity requires us to smile through our tears and deny our pain, and too many of us try to talk others out of theirs. By contrast, the Epistle to the Hebrews tells us that our Lord identified with us so fully in our humanity that he is touched with the very feeling of our infirmities.

Suffering does not necessarily teach endurance, build character, or lead to a mature holiness or Christlikeness. These things can result from suffering, but suffering can also be the great embitterer, the force that leads some to withdraw from life, from love, in a futile attempt to try to protect themselves against more pain. The impact of suffering on our lives, for good or ill, depends largely on our response to it, and in my experience, a creative response is possible only by the grace of God. If we know, really know, that God loves us we can not only begin to accept the difficulties that are part of our lot, but we can begin to transcend them.

The writer Margaret Clarkson was born into a home she describes as loveless and unhappy. From childhood she was afflicted with severe headaches and crippling arthritis. Her responses to her suffering ran the gamut—rage, frustration, despair, even temptation to suicide. But gradually she came to believe that God displays his sovereignty over evil by "using the very suffering that is inherent in evil to assist in the working out of his eternal purpose." In this process he has developed an alchemy greater than that sought by the early chemists who tried to turn base materials like lead into gold. God, says Clarkson in her book *Destined for Glory*, is the only true alchemist, the one who succeeds in the transmutation of evil into good. And God can even transform the pain of our infertility in order to achieve his larger purposes for our lives.

Although I have been speaking personally in these pages, I believe, with Frederick Buechner, that the story of any one of us is to some extent the story of all of us, and I hope readers will find echoes of their own experience here. Beyond that, I hope they will take time to listen carefully to their own lives. As Buechner says near the beginning of the second volume of his graceful autobiography, *Now and Then*, "If God speaks to us at all other than through such official channels as the Bible and the church, then I think that he speaks to us largely through what happens to us, so what I have done . . . in this book . . . is to listen back over what has happened to me—as I hope my readers may listen back over what has happened to them—for the sound, above all else, of his voice."[1]

As I look back over my own experiences over the past few years, I find that the pain of infertility is, more often than not, a faded memory. I am grateful for my life. Grateful for my husband of eighteen years. Grateful for my sense of life as an adventure, which unfolds chapter by chapter. Grateful also for the mercy and forgiveness of God when I fail, and for the knowledge that I can trust him to meet my needs, including the emotional ones. Grateful for friends who are just quietly there. Grateful too for an abundance of small things like the heap of black and white kittens our stray cat, Elspeth, gifted us with two months ago. For the beauty of the natural world—for a recent fall evening when the ground mist was so alight with the scarlet rays of the setting sun, it seemed as though the air was on fire. For the daily comforts of hot water, nourishing food, the shelter of our modest, but comfortable Victorian house, and for the warmth of the woodstove on nights like this one in the cold of a New England December.

It is a tradition in this part of New England to light candles in the front windows of houses from Advent to Epiphany. When I return home from work in the early darkness of these winter evenings, I come off a highway and through a congested business district before slowing down for the villages that lie on my way home. As soon as I begin seeing the Advent lights in the windows, I know I'm close to home and I can feel my body beginning to relax. We're all on our way home. We're all heading for the light and love that await us at the end of our journey. Our Lord said he was going ahead to prepare a place for us, and we can trust him to keep his promise. In the meantime, surely we can also trust him to give us freely what we need along the way. Praise him.

Endnotes

Chapter One

1. Barbara Eck Menning, "The Emotional Needs of Infertile Couples," *Fertility and Sterility* 34 (October 1980) 4:313.

Chapter Three

1. Barbara Eck Menning, "The Emotional Needs of Infertile Couples," *Fertility And Sterility* 34 (October 1980) 4:317.
2. C. S. Lewis, *A Grief Observed* (New York: The Seabury Press, 1961), 7.

Chapter Four

1. Barbara Eck Menning, *A Guide for the Childless Couple* (Englewood Cliffs, N.J.: Prentice Hall, 1977), 18.
2. Robert H. Glass and Ronald J. Ericsson, *Getting Pregnant in the 1980's, New Advances in Infertility Treatment and Sex Preselection* (Berkeley: University of California Press, 1982), 37.
3. John J. Stangel, M.D., *Fertility and Conception: An Essential Guide for Childless Couples* (New York: Paddington Press Ltd., 1979), 87.
4. Barbara Eck Menning, "Common Myths About Infertility," *Resolve* pamphlet.
5. Glass and Ericsson, *Getting Pregnant in the 1980's*, 47.
6. Ibid., 25, 27.
7. Ibid., 6-7.
8. Ibid., 90, 94.

9. Ibid., 90.

10. Madeleine Blais, *They Say You Can't Have a Baby* (New York: W. W. Norton, 1979), 148.

11. C. S. Lewis, *God in the Dock: Essays on Theology and Ethics*, ed. Walter Hooper (Grand Rapids: Wm. B. Eerdmans, 1970), 109-110.

Chapter Five

1. Edith Schaeffer, *Affliction* (Old Tappan, N.J.: Fleming H. Revell, 1978), 212-213.

2. Susan Borg and Judith Lasker, *When Pregnancy Fails: Families Coping With Miscarriage, Stillbirth, and Infant Death* (Boston: Beacon Press, 1981), 8-9.

3. Ibid., 36-37.

4. Rochelle Friedman and Bonnie Gradstein, *Surviving Pregnancy Loss* (Boston: Little Brown and Company, 1982), 13-14.

5. Robert H. Glass and Ronald J. Ericsson, *Getting Pregnant in the 1980's: New Advances in Infertility Treatment and Sex Preselection* (Berkeley: University of California Press, 1982), 58.

6. Ibid., 66.

7. Borg and Lasker, *When Pregnancy Fails*, 163.

8. Friedman and Gradstein, *Surviving Pregnancy Loss*, 38.

Chapter Six

1. Ellen Peck and Judith Senderowitz, *Pronatalism: The Myth of Mom and Apple Pie* (New York: Thomas Y. Crowell, 1974), 156.

2. Mary Perkins Ryan and John Julian Ryan, *Love and Sexuality: A Christian Approach* (New York: Holt, Rinehart and Winston, 1967), 3.

3. Ryan and Ryan, *Love and Sexuality*, 96-97.

4. Walter Trobisch, *I Married You* (San Francisco: Harper & Row, 1971), 20-21.

5. Richard J. Foster, *Freedom of Simplicity* (San Francisco: Harper & Row, 1981), 137.

Chapter Seven

1. Teri Yates is not only the adoptive mother of a little girl, she herself was adopted by an American military family.

Chapter Eight

1. Rosemarie Manganello and Linda Anderson, "The Hannah Syndrome," *Eternity* (December 1977), 25.

2. Timothy Weber, "Empty Quivers," *Eternity* (November 1983), 35- 36.

3. "Making Choices," the 1983 Report of the Alan Guttmacher Institute, a New York-based research group.

4. Manganello and Anderson, "The Hannah Syndrome," *Eternity*, 25.

5. Titus Presler, "Compassion," a sermon preached in Christ Church of Hamilton and Wenham, Massachusetts, July 5, 1983.

Afterthoughts

1. Frederick Buechner, *Now and Then* (New York: Harper and Row, 1983), 3.

Appendix

The resources listed here are among the best available books and services.

INFERTILITY

Organizations

The American Fertility Society
Administrative Office
2140 11th Avenue, South
Suite 200
Birmingham, Alabama 35205
(205) 933-8494

You can write or telephone the Society for the names of the infertility specialists in your area.

Resolve, Inc.
5 Water Street
Arlington, Massachusetts 02174
(617) 643-2424

This national nonprofit organization offers free telephone counseling, referrals to medical services, support groups, and a wealth of excellent literature, including medical fact sheets and a newsletter. Write for a bibliography of publications.

Stepping Stones Ministry
c/o Central Christian Church
2900 North Rock Road
Wichita, Kansas 67226

Supported solely by voluntary contributions, this Christian ministry publishes a free bi-monthly newsletter and serves as a clearinghouse for information on seminars, support groups, and publications.

Books

Anderson, Ann Kiemel. *Taste of Tears, Touch of God*. Nashville, Tenn.: Nelson, 1984.

Barker, Graham, M.D. *Your Search for Fertility*. New York: William Morrow and Company, 1980.

Behrman, S.J., M.D., and Robert W. Kistner, M.D. *Progress in Infertility*. Boston: Little Brown and Company, 2nd edition, 1975.

Decker, Albert, M.D., and Suzanne Loebl. *Why Can't We Have a Baby?* New York: Warner Books, 1978.

Glass, Robert H., and Ronald J. Ericsson. *Getting Pregnant in the 1980's: New Advances in Infertility Treatment and Sex Preselection*. Berkeley, Los Angeles, and London: University of California Press, 1982.

Lifchez, Aaron S., M.D., and Judith A. Fenton. *The Fertility Handbook*. New York: Clarkson N. Potter, 1980.

Menning, Barbara Eck. *Infertility: A Guide for the Childless Couple*. Englewood Cliffs, N.J.: Spectrum Books/Prentice Hall, 1977.

Silber, Sherman J., M.D. *How to Get Pregnant*. New York: Charles Scribner and Sons, 1980.

Stangel, John J., M.D. *Fertility and Conception: An Essential Guide for Childless Couples*. New York and London: Paddington Press Ltd., 1979.

Stigger, Judith. *Coping With Infertility: A Guide for Couples, Families, and Counselors*. Minneapolis, Minn.: Augsburg Publishing House, 1983.

MISCARRIAGE

Borg, Susan, and Judith Lasker. *When Pregnancy Fails: Families Coping With Miscarriage, Stillbirth and Infant Death*. Boston: Beacon Press, 1981.

Friedman, Rochelle, and Bonnie Gradstein. *Surviving Pregnancy Loss*. Boston and New York: Little Brown, 1982.

Williamson, Audrey J. *Miscarriage: Sharing the Grief, Facing the Pain, Healing the Wounds*. New York: Walker and Company, 1987.

"CHILDFREE" LIVING

Ingram, Kristen. *Childless But Not Barren.* Avon, N.J.: Magnificat Press, 1988.

Love, Vicky. *Childless Is Not Less.* Minneapolis, Minn.: Bethany House, 84.

Peck, Ellen, and Judith Senderowitz. *Pronatalism: The Myth of Mom and Apple Pie.* New York: Thomas Y. Crowell, 1974.

Whelan, Elizabeth M. *A Baby? . . . Maybe.* New York: The Bobbs Merrill Company, 1975.

ADOPTION

For a complete list of adoption organizations and resources see *The Adoption Resource Book* and *The Adoption Adviser* (listed below).

Organizations

Bethany Christian Services   Also handles International adoptions.
Central Office
901 Eastern, N.E.
Grand Rapids, MI 49503
(616) 459-6273
(800) 238-4269

National Committee for Adoption
1930 17th St., N.W.
Washington, D.C. 20009
National Adoption Hotline: (202) 328-1200

Organizations Specializing in Foreign Adoptions

International Children's Services
1195 City View
P.O. Box 2880
Eugene, Oregon 97402

Adoptive Families of America
3333 Highway 100 North
Minneapolis, MN 55422
(612) 535-4829

Adoptive Families of America is a national organization for adoptive families. Write for their magazine and bibliography.

Books

Anderson, Ann Kiemel. *And With the Gift Came Laughter.* Wheaton, Ill.: Tyndale House, 1987.

Brandsen, Cheryl Krekes. *A Loving Choice.* Grand Rapids, Mich.: Bethany Christian Services, 1988.

Burgess, Linda Cannon. *The Art of Adoption.* New York: W. W. Norton, 1981.

Carney, Ann. *No More Here and There: Adopting the Older Child.* Chapel Hill, N.C.: The University of North Carolina Press, 1976.

Felker, Donald W. and Evelyn H. *Adoption, Beginning to End.* Grand Rapids, Mich.: Baker Book House, 1987.

Gilman, Lois. *The Adoption Resource Book.* New York: Harper & Row, 1984.

Hunt, Angela. *The Adoption Option.* Wheaton, Ill.: Scripture Press, 1989.

Jewett, Claudia. *Adopting the Older Child.* Boston: Harvard Common Press, 1977.

Kravik, Patricia J. *Adopting Children with Special Needs.* New York: North American Council on Adoptable Children, 1976.

Krementz, Jill. *How it Feels to Be Adopted.* New York: Alfred A. Knopf, 1982.

Martin, Cynthia D. *Beating the Adoption Game.* La Jolla, Calif.: Oaktree Press, 1980.

McNamara, Joan. *The Adoption Adviser,* New York: Hawthorn Books, 1975.

National Committee for Adoption, *Adoption Fact Book.* Washington, D.C.: National Committee for Adoption, 1989.

Plumez, Jacqueline Hornor. *Successful Adoption: A Guide to Finding a Child and Raising a Family.* New York: Crown Publishers, Harmony Books, 1982.

Sorosky, Arthur D., M.D., Annette Baron, M.S.W., and Reuben Pannor, M.S.W. *The Adoption Triangle.* New York: Anchor Press/Doubleday, 1978.

CHRISTIAN PERSPECTIVES ON SUFFERING

Clarkson, Margaret. *Destined for Glory.* Grand Rapids, Mich.: Eerdmans and Marshalls, 1983.

Lewis, C. S. *A Grief Observed.* New York: The Seabury Press, 1961.

_____. *The Problem of Pain.* New York: Macmillan, 1962.

Schaeffer, Edith. *Affliction.* Old Tappan, N.J.: Fleming H. Revell, 1978.

Stigger, Judith. "A Faith on God's Terms," *Coping With Infertility: A Guide for Couples, Families, and Counselors.* Minneapolis, Minn.: Augsburg Publishing House, 1983.

Stott, John R.W. "Suffering and Glory" in *The Cross of Christ.* Downers, Grove, Ill.: InterVarsity Press, 1986.

Yancey, Philip. *Disappointment with God.* Grand Rapids, Mich.: Zondervan, 1989.

_____. *Where Is God When It Hurts?* Grand Rapids, Mich.: Zondervan Publishing House, 1977.

Index